Advocacy

Guest Editor

TERRI GOODMAN, PhD, RN

PERIOPERATIVE NURSING CLINICS

www.periopnursing.theclinics.com

December 2012 • Volume 7 • Number 4

SAUNDERS an imprint of ELSEVIER, Inc.

W.B. SAUNDERS COMPANY

A Division of Elsevier Inc.

1600 John F. Kennedy Boulevard • Suite 1800 • Philadelphia, Pennsylvania 19103-2899

http://www.periopnursing.theclinics.com

PERIOPERATIVE NURSING CLINICS Volume 7, Number 4
December 2012 ISSN 1556-7931, ISBN-13: 978-1-4557-4910-2

Editor: Katie Saunders
Developmental Editor: Donald Mumford

Perioperative Nursing Clinics (ISSN 1556-7931) is published quarterly by Elsevier, 360 Park Avenue South, New York, NY 10010. Months of issue are March, June, September and December. Business and Editorial Offices: 1600 John F. Kennedy Blvd., Suite 1800, Philadelphia, PA 19103-2899. Customer Service Office: 11830 Westline Industrial Drive, St. Louis, MO 63146. Periodicals postage paid at New York, NY and at additional mailing offices. Subscription prices are $132.00 per year (domestic individuals), $224.00 per year (domestic institutions), $65.00.00 per year (domestic students/ residents), $171.00 per year (international individuals), $257.00 per year (international institutions), and $69.00 per year (International students/residents). Foreign air speed delivery is included in all *Clinics* subscription prices. All prices are subject to change without notice. **POSTMASTER:** Send change of address to *Perioperative Nursing Clinics*, Customer Service (orders, claims, online, change of address): Elsevier Periodicals Customer Service, 11830 Westline Industrial Drive, St. Louis, MO 63146. Tel: 1-800-654-2452 (U.S. and Canada). Fax: 314-523-5170. E-mail: journalscustomerservice-usa@elsevier.com (for print support); journalsonlinesupport-usa@elsevier.com (for online support).

Reprints. For copies of 100 or more, of articles in this publication, please contact the Commercial Rights Department, Elsevier Inc., 360 Park Avenue South, New York, NY 10010-1710; Phone: (+1) 212-633-3813; Fax: (+1) 212-462-1935; E-mail: reprints@elsevier.com.

Printed and bound by CPI Group (UK) Ltd, Croydon, CR0 4YY

Transferred to digital print 2012

Contributors

CONSULTING EDITOR

NANCY GIRARD, PhD, RN, FAAN
Nurse Collaborations, Boerne, Texas; Clinical Associate Professor, Acute Nursing Care
Department, University of Texas Health Science Center, San Antonio, Texas

GUEST EDITOR

TERRI GOODMAN, PhD, RN, CNOR
Principal, Terri Goodman and Associates, Dallas, Texas

AUTHORS

CAROL ATHEY, MSN, RN, CNOR
DeWitt School of Nursing Faculty, Stephen F. Austin State University, Nacogdoches,
Texas

ANDREA E. BERNDT, PhD
Family and Community Health Systems Department, School of Nursing, The University of
Texas Health Science Center at San Antonio, San Antonio, Texas

ARACELY LUCENDO DÍAZ, DUE
Perioperative Nurse, Hospital Universitario de Canarias, Ctra. Ofra S/N La Cuesta;
Surgical Nurse, Teacher, Nursing College of Santa Cruz de Tenerife, Tenerife, Canary
Islands, Spain

TIFFANY FACILE, BS, RN, CNOR
Avera McKennan Hospital, Sioux Falls, South Dakota

DONNA A. FORD, MSN, RN-BC, CNOR
Nursing Education Specialist, Department of Nursing and Assistant Professor of Nursing,
College of Medicine, Mayo Clinic, Rochester, Minnesota

PATTI S. GRANT, RN, BSN, MS, CIC
Director, Infection Prevention/Quality, Methodist Hospital for Surgery, Addison, Texas

AMY L. HADER, JD
Director of Government Affairs, AORN, Denver, Colorado

DEBORAH KENDALL-GALLAGHER, PhD, JD, RN
Assistant Professor, Department of Health Restoration & Care Systems Management,
School of Nursing, University of Texas Health Science Center at San Antonio, San Antonio,
Texas

MARY NOUVERTNE KLEIN, RN, MSN, LNFA
Retired

LOLLY LOCKHART, PhD, RN
Health Care Consultant, Pflugerville, Texas

ANN McKENNIS, RN, CNOR(E), CORLN(E)
Retired Perioperative Staff Nurse, The Methodist Hospital, Houston, Texas

REBECCA O'SHEA, MS, RN, OCN, AOCNS, CBCN
Oncology CNS/Navigator/Program Coordinator, Texas Health Presbyterian Hospital, Denton, Texas

JOANNE D. OLIVER, RN, BSN, CNOR
Owner/CEO, Healthcare Resources, Houston, Texas

ROSEMARY K. RUSHMER, PhD
School of Health and Social Care, Teesside University, Middlesbrough, Yorkshire, United Kingdom

EVELYN SWENSON-BRITT, PhD, RN
Center for Excellence in Patient Care, University Health System, San Antonio, Texas

KATHRYN M. TART, EdD, MSN, BA
Founding Dean and Professor, School of Nursing, University of Houston Victoria, Victoria, Texas

MIKE THOMAS, RN, MA, BSN, CNOR, MLSSBB
Director, Surgical Services, Baylor Regional Medical Center, Plano, Texas

MICHAEL VAN DOREN, MSN, RN, CARN
Program Director, Texas Peer Assistance Program for Nurses, Austin, Texas

JAMES H. WILLMANN, JD
Department of Governmental Affairs, Texas Nurses Association, Austin, Texas

CINDY DIAMOND ZOLNIEREK, PhD(c), MSN, RN
Assistant Professor, St. David's School of Nursing, Texas State University; Doctoral Candidate, School of Nursing, University of Texas at Austin

Contents

Public policy decisions directly affect nurses and their patients. Participating in the legislative process is one of the most, if not the most, significant ways in which nurses can affect public policy. If nurses do not participate, important public policy decisions affecting nurses, nursing practice, and patients are made without nursing input. Nurses are more likely to be effective and successful in participating in the legislative process by following certain principles which include understanding how the legislative process works, understanding the role of negotiation and compromise, and having an effective decision-making process.

The most significant action that nurses can take to manage the changing health care environment is to advocate for patients, for the profession of nursing, and for each other. The Institute of Medicine (IOM) report *To Err is Human* started a groundswell of concern for patient safety. The IOM then released their report *Keeping Patients Safe: Transforming the Work Environment of Nurses*, acknowledging that nurses have a major impact on patient safety. This article argues for a culture of safety in the nursing workplace.

Advocacy can be defined as "the act of pleading or supporting"; to advocate is to "plead in favor of." Nurse advocacy may be thought of as "speaking out and speaking for patients." But how does advocacy occur in nursing practice? How does an individual nurse provide a voice on behalf of patients that is heard? This article reviews the concept of patient advocacy and the role of nurses. Challenges to advocacy activities are presented and strategies for effective advocacy practice are discussed.

There are 6 levels through which an individual nurse can advocate for patients, health care, and the nursing profession. By cultivating relationships, expressing positions clearly and precisely, and being dependable and involved in the decision-making environment, a nurse can be an influential advocate. This article discusses the levels of advocacy and describes the steps and behaviors that lead to a position of influence.

Joanne D. Oliver

Nurses must actively participate in influencing the future of health care and the nursing profession. Involvement in the legislative process is an effective way to influence access to health care, health care costs, and the role of nursing in the health care environment. Read and research the legislation being presented; formulate a personal plan for your own involvement. Know your legislators and communicate with them consistently. As informed, committed, and enthusiastic supporters of legislation that furthers our objectives, 3.1 million registered nurses can educate and influence legislators and promote the future in which we believe.

SECTION II: Advocating for Nurses and Patients

Mike Thomas

A culture of safety and advocacy is the most effective environment in which to address workplace challenges successfully and deliver outstanding, safe patient care. A safe or just culture encourages employees to be vigilant, to identify and examine close calls to prevent errors. Such a culture emphasizes patient safety, retains employees, curbs spiraling healthcare costs, and meets regulatory and patient expectations of care.

Patti S. Grant

This article proposes a nursing evidence-based practice (EBP) starter kit for smaller health care facilities, with a novel triangular approach to nursing EBP to consider strength of evidence, time management, and a culture of safety. Internet-based references are suggested for this novel EBP triangular approach. Safety dialogue and references for nurse empowerment toward furthering safety culture are suggested. The application of Stephen R. Covey's "7 Habits" Circle of Influence and Time Management Matrix toward implementation of nursing EBP is proposed.

Andrea E. Berndt, Evelyn Swenson-Britt, and Rosemary K. Rushmer

This article considers barriers to nurses' collective learning in perioperative units and suggests the development of learning practice communities as a potential solution. Several characteristics of learning practice communities are identified and strategies to encourage their development in perioperative units are proposed.

Donna A. Ford

Perioperative nurses are patient advocates in the patient/nurse relationship, but this advocacy role extends much further. Perioperative nurses can advocate for their collective patients through professional nursing association membership, continually updating their professional knowledge, supporting their professional nursing association through participation, and the use of patient safety and workplace safety resources. Perioperative nurses serve as advocates to their patients through various activities in professional nursing associations, which provide support through practice resources, education, and legislative activities. Advocacy between perioperative nurses and professional nursing associations is symbiotic, and serves to improve the quality of patient care and the profession of nursing.

Amy L. Hader

The Association of periOperative Registered Nurses (AORN) advocates for the 160,000 perioperative nurses practicing in the United States. AORN establishes practice recommendations and legislative priorities for its 40,000 members and the perioperative nursing field in general.

Tiffany Facile

The current and future generations of nurses will replace the aging perioperative workforce. New nurses must be welcomed into the operating room and their success as perioperative team members facilitated. Old habits, strong personalities, and unprofessional bullying must not occur without opposition. Professionals need to support every member of their surgical teams, embrace process changes, learn from failures, and celebrate successes. A concerted effort must be made to change so-called eating our young behaviors into practices that empower our new perioperative nurses.

SECTION III: Advocating for Specific Patient Populations

Michael Van Doren

Peer assistance programs for nurses facilitate preservation of a nursing license and return to work for nurses with substance use or psychiatric disorders who are in recovery. Peer assistance advocates are volunteer nurses who are pursuing education and training to provide one-to-one support for nurses participating in the program. Peer assistance advocates also provide education to nursing colleagues and employers of program participants.

> Nurses advocating for older patients can help them deal effectively with the maze of insensitive territory, endless questions, and unexplained testing. As the number of elderly patients increases, there is a greater need for experience in gerontology in all medical and nursing specialties. Good preoperative planning includes an effective transition of care from the hospital to home, reducing the potential for complications and rehospitalization. Older adults are particularly sensitive to medications, which must be aggressively reviewed so that unnecessary drugs are eliminated and dosages are adjusted for optimal effect.

> This article presents the author's recommendations to perioperative managers and caregivers for overcoming the barriers to sensitive and appropriate care of pediatric patients in an adult environment. Preparation for this article included an extensive literature search including the United Nations "Convention on the Rights of the Child," which provides a comprehensive framework of rights that facilitates a holistic approach to promote the well-being of children. Documents from the World Health Organization, UNICEF, and the European Union also speak to the specialized care to which patients under 19 are entitled.

> Advances in treatment options have made cancer a more controllable disease. How the patient and family are told about a cancer diagnosis and how they are supported through treatment and long-term follow-up are critical to adherence and compliance. As the number of cancer survivors increases, their unique needs, both immediate and long-term, have become central to nurses' advocacy role.

> Laryngectomees (people with permanent tracheal stomas as a result of larynx removal) face major life changes: in their body image, how they communicate because they are unable to talk, and how they eat. Advocating for laryngectomees facing this difficult challenge facilitates a more rapid adjustment to a different but manageable lifestyle. With the support of nurse advocates, laryngectomee patients can learn to advocate for themselves.

Special Feature Article

> March 2012 marked the second anniversary of the Affordable Care Act (ACA), landmark legislation designed to transform health care delivery in

the United States. Understanding how the ACA will impact care delivered in the hospital setting is essential for perioperative nurses if they are to influence and lead change to improve the quality, efficiency, and effectiveness of care.

x

Advocacy

PERIOPERATIVE NURSING CLINICS

We regret to announce that this issue, December 2012, will mark the final issue of this series, as *Perioperative Nursing Clinics* ceases publication.

Perioperative Nursing Clinics issues maintained a high level of quality in content, relevant topics and adept authors throughout its 2006–2012 print run.

Since September 2008, Consulting Editor, Nancy Girard, PhD, RN, FAAN, has led the series capably and gracefully. She has been a treasured collaborator and expert for the series, as well as someone I have come to consider a friend.

I will truly miss working with Nancy, and all of the talented Guest Editors and authors who I have had the pleasure of collaborating with on the series.

Sincerely,

Katie Saunders

Katie Saunders, Editor

DOWNLOAD
Free App!

Review Articles
THE CLINICS

NOW AVAILABLE FOR YOUR iPhone and iPad

Preface

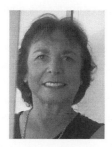

Terri Goodman, PhD, RN, CNOR
Guest Editor

To advocate is *"to support or recommend publicly; to plead for or speak in favor of."*[1] When we think of the nurse as an advocate, we think first of stepping up to protect a patient's rights or to prevent an act that could jeopardize the patient's safety. In fact, nurses advocate in many arenas and in many different ways. This issue of *Perioperative Nursing Clinics* explores the broad spectrum of advocacy in nursing. In addition to advocating for individual patients, nurses advocate for all patients, for specific patient populations, for our nursing colleagues, for the specialty of perioperative nursing, and for the profession of nursing.

To advocate is to participate actively in achieving an outcome. The more strongly a nurse believes in the importance and the "rightness" of an issue, the more enthusiastically he or she will participate in advocating to achieve the desired outcome; the more risks the nurse will be willing to face that are sometimes associated with the process. To stand up and speak out in favor of something suggests that there may be opposition to that position. Telling a surgeon or anesthesiologist that the patient's procedure should be postponed is risky; it involves disrupting individual schedules, the OR schedule, and the patient's and family's schedule and may have other negative consequences. However, if the nurse feels strongly that postponing the procedure is the right thing to do, he or she is likely to advocate actively in the face of opposition and risk personal consequences in pursuit of the desired outcome.

The environment in which the nurse practices will have a significant impact on both the nurse's willingness to advocate and the potential for success. A *Just Culture* or *Culture of Safety* is one in which individuals are encouraged to identify potentially harmful situations, to admit mistakes or near misses, and to speak up to prevent negative outcomes without fear of censure or retaliation. Such environments are the reflection of the values at the highest level of the organization and cannot be sustained without the support of the organization's leaders. Our nation's health care organizations are working toward this type of environment, but old habits are hard to break, and the *shame and blame* culture is still prevalent. Health care employees are not powerless; they can influence an organization's evolution toward a *Just Culture*.

Articles in this issue demonstrate that nurses, individually and collectively, have both the responsibility and the opportunity to influence health care in our country.

Perioperative Nursing Clinics 7 (2012) xi–xii
http://dx.doi.org/10.1016/j.cpen.2012.09.002
1556-7931/12/$ – see front matter © 2012 Elsevier Inc. All rights reserved.

Nurses have unlimited opportunities to advocate for what they believe to be right and in the best interests of patients, the nursing profession, and our country's health care environment, including the responsibility and opportunity to advocate for the environment that permits us to speak up without fear of reprisal.

Terri Goodman, PhD, RN, CNOR
Terri Goodman and Associates
Dallas, TX 75229, USA

E-mail address:
terrigoodman@sbcglobal.net

REFERENCE

1. Dictionary.com.   http://dictionary.reference.com/browse/advocate.   Accessed September 12, 2012.

The Nurse as Advocate

Advocating for Nursing through Public Policy

James H. Willmann, JD

KEYWORDS

• Advocacy • Public policy • Legislative process

KEY POINTS

• Public policy decisions directly affect nurses and their patients.
• Participating in the legislative process is one of the most, if not the most, significant ways in which nurses can affect public policy.
• If nurses do not participate, important public policy decisions affecting nurses, nursing practice, and patients are made without nursing input.
• Nurses are more likely to be effective and successful in participating in the legislative process by following certain principles which include understanding how the legislative process works, understanding the role of negotiation and compromise, and having an effective decision-making process.

INTRODUCTION

The US Capitol Building in Washington, DC and the Texas Capitol Building in Austin, Texas may seem distant from the day-to-day practice of nurses. However, both are places where significant public policy decisions are made (or not made) that affect nurses and nursing practice. An obvious example of how public policy affects nursing is health care financing, because so much of health care is now financed through governmental programs such as Medicare and Medicaid. In Texas, more than 55% of births are paid by Medicaid.[1] Public policy decisions about how these programs operate (who is covered, what services are covered, and what reimbursement rates are) directly affect significant patient populations and the nurses who care for those populations.

This article explores the concept of advocating for nurses and the nursing profession through affecting public policy. Because participating in the legislative process is one of the most, if not the most, significant ways in which nurses can affect public policy, this article focuses on affecting public policy through the legislative process.

Department of Governmental Affairs, Texas Nurses Association, 7600 Burnet Road, #440, Austin, TX 78757, USA
E-mail address: jwillmann@texasnurses.org

[1] Texas Health and Human Services Commission presentation January 2011 titled *Medicaid and Healthy Babies*.

Perioperative Nursing Clinics 7 (2012) 367–374
http://dx.doi.org/10.1016/j.cpen.2012.08.014
1556-7931/12/$ – see front matter © 2012 Published by Elsevier Inc.

NURSING AND THE LEGISLATIVE PROCESS

A preliminary question that may be asked by some nurses is "Why should nurses and nursing be involved in trying to affect setting public policy through the legislative process?" It certainly would be easier for nurses simply to care for their patients and not have to deal with the hassle of trying to affect what happens in Washington, DC, Austin, Texas, the other 49 state capitals, or the District of Columbia.

There are several valid reasons for nursing to participate in public policy making through the legislative process. First, nurses not being involved does not mean that public policy decisions affecting nursing and nurses are not made. They are! Rather, nursing's not participating simply means policy decisions are made without nursing input and, in many cases, by persons who do not understand nursing and the role of nurses in the health care system. This situation should be a concern for nurses, not only for themselves but also for their patients.

The issue is not so much that the decisions are made or influenced by individuals who are not supportive of nursing or who may wish to harm nurses (although that is sometimes the case); the issue is that decisions are made by individuals who do not understand nursing and the negative consequences (albeit unintended) that their decisions may have on nursing and patients. An example of an unintended consequence is legislation that was seriously considered by the Texas Legislature[2] in 2011. The legislation would have required the Texas Medical Board to disclose to a physician reported to the board the identity of the person who reported that physician. The only exception was when the physician was reported by a patient or a member of the patient's family. Disclosing the person's identity was characterized as a good public policy because it would discourage groundless complaints against physicians.

The legislation was passing without serious opposition until nursing initiated a campaign against the proposal because of the chilling effect that it would have on nurses reporting physicians whom they believed were practicing below the acceptable standard of care. Nursing pointed out that retaliation against a nurse who reports a physician was not an unfounded fear given what had just happened to 2 nurses in Winkler County, Texas, whose employment was terminated and who were criminally indicted as a result of reporting a physician to the Texas Medical Board. Nursing also pointed out that physicians are often in a position to retaliate directly or indirectly against a nurse who reports them. Because nurses were proactive and participated in the legislative process, the legislation was amended to specifically protect the confidentiality of nurses who report physicians.

A second reason for nursing to be involved in affecting public policy through the legislative process is that nurses and their patients have benefited from active participation in the legislative process. (**Box 1**) lists some legislative accomplishments in Texas that would be unlikely to have occurred without nursing being involved. Certainly, nurses in Texas and their patients are better off because of these legislative accomplishments.

A third, and perhaps the most important reason that nursing and nurses should be involved in public policy making is that the perspective of nursing is essential. Nursing is consistently recognized as the most trusted profession in the nation.[3] Nurses are

---

[2] Because the author, as Director of Governmental Affairs for the Texas Nurses Association, is most familiar with public advocacy for nursing at the Texas Legislature, the examples in this article reflect that experience.
[3] In 2011, Gallup's annual poll on trustworthy professions showed nursing at the top for the 12th time in the 13 years the poll had listed nursing as an option.

> **Box 1**
> **Examples of legislative accomplishments in Texas as a result of nursing involvement**
>
> 1. Protection from retaliation for nurses who engage in protected patient advocacy activities
> 2. Peer review for nurses by a committee of their peers
> 3. Peer assistance for nurses who are experiencing problems with chemical dependency and mental illness
> 4. Recognition of the Registered Nurse First Assistant (RNFA) role and the Circulating RN role in the operating room (OR)
> 5. Nurse staffing committees as standing hospital committees that report to the hospital governing board
> 6. Safe patient handling
> 7. Protection for the title "nurse"
> 8. Prescriptive authority for Advanced Practice RNs (APRNs)

one of the most patient-centered of the health care professions. Patients benefit when the nursing perspective is present when public policy decisions are made. This reason alone should be ample justification for nurses and nursing to expend the resources needed to effectively participate in the legislative process.

Addressing public policy through the legislative process is often the only way to affect change for the entire nursing profession or at least a significant segment of the profession (eg, educators, RNFAs, APRNs). Change at the individual facility or local level seldom affects nurses other than those who practice at that facility. Even changes in a large multifacility system affect only the nurses who work within that system. However, changes at the level of state legislation affect all nurses in the state or at least all nurses in a particular practice setting.

EFFECTIVE PARTICIPATION

Nurses not only want to participate in the process, they want to be successful in affecting public policy. One of the first steps is to determine whether an issue is susceptible to a legislative solution. Some issues are best resolved through legislation; others can be addressed more effectively with a nonlegislative solution. For example, increasing wages for nurses is not likely to be susceptible to a legislative solution. Legislators do not want to get involved in setting wages for a predominately privately employed profession. One reason for avoiding such legislation is that it interferes with the free enterprise system. Another equally important motivation is that it sets an undesirable precedent. If the legislature sets wages for the nursing profession, other professions expect the same attention to their wages. Consequently, expending resources on legislation to increase wages for nurses is unlikely to be a productive use of those resources.

On the other hand, expanding prescriptive authority for APRNs can be accomplished only through the legislative process because it involves removing legal barriers (professional licensing laws and pharmacy laws about who can prescribe) that currently limit the extent to which APRNs can prescribe. Unless the law is changed to remove or reduce existing barriers, APRNs' authority to prescribe will not expand. Hence, the only solution is a legislative solution.

There are also issues that may be susceptible to both a legislative and nonlegislative solution. In such cases, the impact of the legislation is likely to address a broader population. One example is protecting nurses from retaliation for advocating for patients.

Nurses may successfully advocate for adequate protections at the individual facility level or even at the system level in multifacility systems. However, even in the latter, only the nurses who practice within that system have the benefit of those protections. Even if nurses who practice at other facilities or within other systems are successful in also getting protections adopted, the protections are likely to differ in some respects from those adopted by other facilities and systems. A consistent, uniform set of patient advocacy protections that cover all nurses almost certainly requires legislation.

An important question is "How does nursing bring to bear the resources needed to participate effectively in the legislative process?" The short answer is that the participation of nursing in the legislative process is almost always through a nursing association, particularly if they want to address multiple issues over an extended period. Individual nurses cannot marshal the resources to participate effectively. Participation in multiorganization coalitions is frequently the most effective way for nursing organizations to participate. For broad-based health policy issues such as immunizations, prenatal care, uninsured children, and public health initiatives, nursing usually participates in coalitions with nonnursing groups, including both health care organizations and consumer advocacy groups.

Even on nursing issues, it is often advantageous for nursing organizations to come together as a coalition. Since the mid-1990s, nursing organizations in Texas have participated in the Nursing Legislative Agenda Coalition (NLAC) (**Box 2**) to develop and support a common legislative agenda. Each organization has its own legislative

---

Box 2
Nursing Legislative Agenda Coalition (NLAC)

Hosted by the Texas Nurses Association, the NLAC meets before each legislative session to develop and support a common nursing agenda. Currently NLAC comprises the following nursing organizations.

Texas Nurses Association

Texas Council of Perioperative Registered Nurses

Texas RNFA Network

Association of periOperative Registered Nurses–Houston

Texas Association of Nurses Anesthetists

Coalition for Nurses in Advanced Practice

Texas Nurse Practitioners

Association of Women's Health, Obstetrics and Neonatal Nurses

Texas Emergency Nurses Association

Society of Otorhinolaryngology and Head and Neck Nurses–Houston

Houston Chapter of Oncology Nursing Society

Texas School Nurses' Organization

Texas Organization of Nurse Executives

Houston Organization of Nurse Executives

Licensed Vocational Nurses Association of Texas

Texas Association of Deans and Directors of Professional Nursing Programs

Texas Organization of Baccalaureate and Graduate Nurse Educators

Texas Organization for Associate Degree Nursing Educators

Texas Nursing Students' Association

priorities. They have the opportunity to educate their colleagues about their issues and gain their support. This collaboration allows all of the member organizations to claim that an issue is supported by all of the major nursing organizations in Texas, a powerful asset when communicating with legislators. Even when nursing is pursuing a nursing initiative, collaborating with nonnursing stakeholders strengthens the position of nursing.

It is essential to understand the following 3 rules, or principles, about participating effectively in the legislative process.

1. "Understand how the legislative process works." In most legislatures, there are points in the process when less than a majority can prevent legislation from moving forward. For example, a committee chair determines when a bill receives a hearing. This single individual can block a bill by delaying until there is insufficient time for it to be passed. There may be a procedural rule that permits fewer than most legislators to block a bill from being voted on. This rule recognizes that even when the votes are there to pass a bill, it may still not pass. Because of this rule, negotiation and compromise with other stakeholders are frequently critical to passing legislation. Legislative sessions are shorter than they seem. In the first weeks, time is devoted to infrastructure needs such as committee appointments; discussing and voting on legislative issues occur later in the session. Each bill is assigned to a committee, where it can be addressed expediently or allowed to languish until it is too late to be heard and voted on by legislators. It is imperative to develop good relationships and consistent communication with the legislators on the committees dealing with the initiatives in which nurses are interested.
2. "Don't let the desire for the perfect prevent doing good." The legislative process encourages negotiation and compromise. In the process of give and take, seldom does either side get everything it wants. However, nurses often feel passionate about their issues. For example, no nurse should have to fear retaliation for advocating for patients. This situation can make it difficult for nurses to view a compromise as a good outcome, even if it is a significant improvement over existing law.
3. "An effective decision-making process is critical." Despite being a generally slow and deliberate process overall, the legislative process moves quickly at times and effective participation requires the ability to make decisions quickly. A membership organization that has to go back to its full membership to make or change a decision is likely to find itself the victim of lost opportunities. Appoint and empower spokespersons to make decisions quickly on behalf of the organization. To be truly effective, this process is likely to require permitting a small group of individuals, or in some limited circumstances, a single individual, to make important decisions. Perhaps the organization's governmental affairs committee or board of directors can be empowered to make decisions. If that is too large a group for a rapid response, an executive committee or the president and executive director might be appropriate spokespersons. To be successful in the unusual circumstance when an immediate decision is necessary to avoid a lost opportunity, a group may need to empower whoever is at the table at the time the decision is made to speak for the group. Other conditions necessary for this process to work are (1) that the issue be thoroughly vetted by the organization so that the individuals making the decision can represent the values and interests of the members and (2) that membership trust the individuals making the decision.

CASE STUDIES

The following 3 cases show some of the principles and considerations for effective participation.

Case Study 1: Protecting the Nurse's Role as Patient Advocate

One of the most important roles that nurses play is that of patient advocate. Nurses spend more time at the bedside with patients than any other health professional and frequently are in the best position to advocate for the patient. Few would question the concept that nurses should be able to advocate for their patients without fear of retaliation. The policy question is how best to implement that principle. Several considerations come to mind that make a legislative solution the preferred approach. First, the goal is that all nurses in all settings enjoy patient advocacy protections. Second, patient advocacy protections for nurses should be uniform across all practice settings and should not vary by facility or practice setting. One of the advantages of addressing issues through public policy is that the policy normally applies uniformly to the entire profession and all practice settings. Conversely, addressing patient advocacy protections on a facility-by-facility basis neither produces protections for all nurses nor is it likely to provide uniform protections among facilities. Hence, legislation is needed to protect the role of all RNs as patient advocates. However, achieving an optimal legislative solution is not necessarily easy; seldom does one achieve everything desired all at once or on the first attempt.

In Texas, the effort to ensure patient advocacy protections for nurses has spanned nearly 25 years and the effort is not yet completed. The initial step was taken in 1987, when protection for nurses who reported nurses to the nursing board and other practitioners to their respective licensing boards was passed. In subsequent legislative sessions, protection has been extended to reporting licensed health care facilities as well as individual practitioners to the appropriate licensing board. Protection was then expanded to include not only the reporting of unsafe care to a licensing board but also the reporting or raising of patient care concerns internally within the facilities. Texas also enacted what is referred to as Safe Harbor Nursing Peer Review. This policy provides a mechanism for a nurse in an untenable position (eg, caring for too many patients or assigned to a task for which they do not feel competent) to implement safe harbor and seek an advisory opinion from a nursing peer review committee as to what a nurse's duty is to the patient in that particular situation. The nurse is afforded protection both from retaliatory action by the facility/employer for requesting the review and also from the Board of Nursing for accepting the assignment pending the nursing peer review committee's determination. For example, it is seldom in the patient's best interest for a nurse questioning the adequacy of staffing to not accept an assignment because that simply means 1 nurse fewer to care for the patient. However, by implementing the Safe Harbor Nursing Peer Review process, the situation that the nurse believed was unsafe comes under review and the nurse does not have to fear retaliation for pointing it out.

Protecting the patient advocacy role of nurses means more than just making retaliation illegal. There must also be a remedy for the nurse who is retaliated against. One remedy is to subject the practitioner or facility retaliating against the nurse to administrative action by their licensing agency. Although this is an important remedy and one that Texas law provides, it is not a remedy that is likely to make the nurse satisfied if their employment has been terminated or they have been otherwise disciplined by the employer. Termination and other disciplinary action usually result not only in direct economic harm to the nurse but also noneconomic harm such as mental anguish and potentially tarnished reputation. To provide the nurse with a remedy for this type of harm, Texas law was amended to give the nurse the right to file a civil lawsuit to recover compensation for these types of damages.

However, adequate protection for all nurses has yet to be fully realized because of the doctrine of sovereign immunity, meaning that a governmental entity cannot be sued for damages unless Congress or the state legislature passes a law waiving sovereign immunity. Consequently, publicly employed nurses in Texas who work in public hospitals or other public health care facilities do not have the same right as their privately employed colleagues to file a lawsuit for damages, except to the extent afforded all other public employees in Texas. Public employees in Texas do have some protections, but only when retaliated against for making a report to a licensing or regulatory agency. Although public hospitals have expressed support for the legislation, nursing has been unsuccessful in the past 2 legislative sessions to secure a waiver of sovereign immunity, so publicly employed nurses who are retaliated against for reporting patient care concerns within the facility have the same right to file a civil lawsuit for damages as privately employed nurses. The opposition to the legislation has come from county governments and legislators, who philosophically oppose any legislation that expands their exposure to a lawsuit.

Case Study 2: RNFAs, Non-RNFAs, and Surgical Technologists

Because surgery is normally characterized as a medical act, questions arose in Texas whether the RNFA, when assisting with surgery, was practicing under their license or practicing under the delegated authority of the surgeon. Issues had also arisen about whether insurers could refuse to reimburse RNFAs for first assisting even although they would reimburse a physician who first assists. To address these issues, nursing organizations representing RNFAs and OR nurses joined with other nursing organizations to initiate legislation to amend the Texas Nursing Practice Act to recognize that when RNFAs assist at surgery, they are practicing under their nursing license. The legislation also amended the Texas Insurance Code to require RNFAs be reimbursed for their services.

A related issue in Texas involved subsequent initiatives by surgical assistants who were not nurses and surgical technologists to be licensed or otherwise recognized and regulated by the State of Texas. Both initiatives involved aspects that nursing regarded as harmful to patients and to nursing. These issues included the appropriate education and training of individuals who first assist, protecting the nurse in the scrub role, ensuring the role of the circulating RN in overseeing the OR, the scope of practice of the surgical technologist, and the relationship of the surgical technologist to the circulating RN. Through effective involvement in the legislative process, nursing was able to secure a satisfactory resolution of these issues. However, these initiatives are good examples of public policy changes that affect nursing being initiated by entities other than nursing. Nurses must be vigilant and actively involved in the legislative process to ensure that legislation affecting nurses and their patients is identified and addressed productively.

Case Study 3: Prescriptive Authority for APRNs

APRNs in every state have addressed this issue. The initiative to achieve prescriptive authority for APRNs in Texas has been a long and ongoing process, showing that achieving a significant legislative change is not likely to occur all at once, but rather through a series of advances over time. The APRN prescriptive authority initiative also shows that one's goal may change over time.

In the late 1970s, when nursing first started seeking recognition for APRNs and greater authority for them to practice to the extent of the education and experience, there was no talk of autonomous prescriptive authority, even as a desired goal. The need for prescriptive authority did not emerge until the late 1980s or early 1990s.

In 1981, Texas APRNs achieved the right to practice under "standing delegation orders," which permitted them to see and treat patients without being first seen by a physician. In 1989, APRNs achieved prescriptive authority at sites serving medically underserved populations, which was extended to other sites in 1995. The authority to prescribe controlled substances schedules III to V was achieved in 2003, which was followed by a 4-year (2 legislative sessions)[4] moratorium on expansion of scope of practice. In the following 2 sessions (2009 and 2011), there were unsuccessful initiatives to achieve autonomous practice.

In preparation for the 2013 session, the nursing organizations representing APRNs convened an APRN Roundtable to develop the 2013 APRN prescriptive authority initiative. Discussions were held with key nonnursing stakeholders and legislators about what they believed might be politically viable initiatives. As a result of this process, nursing has decided to pursue a "collaborative prescriptive authority agreement" model, which 17 states have adopted.[5] The issue of APRN prescriptive authority shows that one of the difficulties that can be encountered in affecting public policy is significant opposition by a group (in this case medical associations) with considerable resources. The APRN groups are members of NLAC and have the support of the member organizations.

SUMMARY

Knowledge of the legislative process and active participation are essential to protecting the rights of nurses and patients. Understanding that an outcome, given the political and cultural environment, might best be achieved in increments over several legislative sessions can help to craft successful initiatives. Collaboration is a powerful tool; initiatives with broad support are more attractive to legislators. Consistent involvement in public policy is necessary to identify issues that have an impact on nurses, the nursing profession, and patients, even when the issues are initiated by nonnursing groups.

---

[4] Texas has biennial sessions, which last for 140 days (January–May) each odd-numbered year. Special sessions may be called, but they are normally called only to address major state issues such as the budget, and legislative redistricting that were unable to be resolved during the regular 140-day session.

[5] Another 18 states plus the District of Columbia have adopted autonomous practice.

Advocacy Now: A Perioperative Imperative

Lolly Lockhart, PhD, RN

KEYWORDS

- Nurse advocacy • Nurse leadership • Patient safety • Nurse safety
- Culture of safety • Code for nurses

KEY POINTS

- The most significant action that nurses can take to manage the changing health care environment is to advocate for patients, for the profession of nursing, and for each other.
- The Institute of Medicine (IOM) report *To Err is Human* started a groundswell of concern for patient safety.
- The IOM then released their report *Keeping Patients Safe: Transforming the Work Environment of Nurses* acknowledging that nurses have a major impact on patient safety.

Our world, the United States, health care, and nursing are all at "tipping points," facing chaos with its constant and unpredictable change. To survive and thrive in this complex environment, nurses have to change the way they relate to one another and how they do business. The most significant action that nurses, individually and collectively, can take to manage the chaos is to engage in dialogue, advocating for patients, for the profession of nursing, and for each other. The time is ripe for nurses to move to the forefront and have a positive impact on the health care system and nursing. Nurses must be prepared to face opposition, and possibly retaliation, but they must accept the challenge.

The Institute of Medicine (IOM) report *To Err is Human: Building a Safer Health System* (2000)[1] started a groundswell of concern for patient safety that quickly led the IOM to release their report *Keeping Patients Safe: Transforming the Work Environment of Nurses* (KPS) (2004),[2] acknowledging that nurses and the environment in which we practice have a major impact on patient safety. KPS made several excellent recommendations that have yet to be realized. First, those who practice in health care must change their approach to decision making from transactional (top down) to transformational (shared governance). The American Nurses Credentialing Center's (ANCC) *Magnet Designation and Pathways to Excellence*[3] recognition programs have helped make some advances in this change, with much left to be done in both clinical settings and in academia. Second, we must create in our working and practice environments a Culture of Safety or a Just Culture.

3520 Killingsworth Lane, Pflugerville, TX 78660, USA
E-mail address: Lollylock@gmail.com

Perioperative Nursing Clinics 7 (2012) 375–377
http://dx.doi.org/10.1016/j.cpen.2012.08.004   **periopnursing.theclinics.com**
1556-7931/12/$ – see front matter © 2012 Published by Elsevier Inc.

We hear stories of nurses stepping out and making a difference by stopping a surgeon from wearing latex gloves to perform surgery on a patient with latex allergy, yet we also hear of an experienced neonatal intensive care nurse, distracted in preparing a medication, who gave an overdose to an infant. Even though the nurse immediately reported her error, she was disciplined and became so distraught with the punitive response that she committed suicide. We have a long way to go.

In KPS, a Culture of Safety recognizes first that the majority of errors are created by systemic organizational defects in work processes; second, that the top leadership supports staff; and finally, that staff experience opportunities for continuous learning. In a Just Culture an individual faces no threat of retaliation for speaking up. For patients' safety, nurses are encouraged to report their own errors and the errors of others, as well as "near misses," without fear of retaliation or facing the old "shame and blame" response. Safety for patients and nurses must be a priority.

Successfully managing the challenge of this chaotic environment is the key to our future! It is not optional. The American Nurses Association Bill of Rights for Registered Nurses (2001)[4] supports nurses' advocating for themselves and for other nurses, as well as advocating for those whom we serve. We need to do a "cultural assessment" in our work environments, to determine whether our leadership had transitioned from a transactional to transformational culture. Are nurses at all levels in an organization effectively engaged in the decision-making/problem-solving process? Are communications and relationships among nurses and other health care professionals transparent when they address potential and actual adverse events concerning patients? We need nurse advocacy throughout the environment: within our leadership, in middle management, and within the ranks of direct care nurses.

The 2010 IOM report, *The Future of Nursing* (FON),[5] presents an opportunity for nurses to address the complexity effectively and participate in the change that is currently taking place. Among the FON recommendations are (1) expanding opportunities for nurses to lead and diffuse collaborative improvement efforts, and (2) to prepare and enable nurses to lead change to advance health. Nurses are challenged to move to the forefront and be leaders in the current restructuring of the American health care system. Nurses must accept the challenge to introduce transformational leadership and advocacy into all areas of nursing and health care. Nurses must see that a Culture of Safety and a Just Culture are established wherever they work: in clinical practice and in academia. In the past, nurses have not been able to move together effectively, but in our current environment of chaos and constant change, there is an opportunity to engage and make a significant impact. It is time for nurses to put aside differences and take advantage of this opportunity.

Nurses must work to ensure that workplaces are managed with transformational processes that promote transparent sharing and problem solving in a Culture of Safety. Nurses must encourage one another to step out of their comfort zones and be willing to lead the change. The *Interpretive Guidelines to the ANA Code for Nurses* (2010)[6] warn us that when nurses advocate for patient safety or for one another, they are indeed advocating against something, someone, or the "system." Advocacy can be an easy or a challenging process, depending on the circumstances and the culture in place. No matter the situation, nurses must be prepared to accept the challenge, face opposition, and address retaliation. There are resources in place to protect nurses to advocate for their patients, their colleagues, their profession, and for themselves.

REFERENCES

1. Institute of Medicine. (200). To err is human. Washington, DC: National Academy Press. Available at: www.nap.edu.

2. Institute of Medicine. Keeping patient safe: transforming the work environment for nurses. Washington, DC: National Academy Press; 2004. Available at: www.nap.edu.
3. CCNE Magnet and pathways to excellence. Available at: http://nursecredentialing. org/magnet.aspx http://nursecredentialing.org/pathway.aspx.
4. American Nurses Association. ANA bill of rights for registered nurses. American Nurses Association; 2001.
5. Institute of Medicine. The future of nursing: leading change, advancing health. Washington, DC: National Academy Press; 2010. Available at: www.nap.edu.
6. American Nurses Association. Code of ethics for nurses with interpretive guidelines. American Nurses Association; 2010.

Beyond Rhetoric
Supporting Patient Advocacy in Nursing Practice

Cindy Diamond Zolnierek, PhD(c), MSN, RN[a,b,*]

KEYWORDS

- Patient advocacy • Nursing practice • Quality standards

KEY POINTS

- Nurses play a protective role for patients by identifying and raising concerns so that issues can be evaluated and addressed.
- The public depends on such patient advocacy efforts to ensure care achieves safety and quality standards.
- Patient advocacy by nurses involves speaking out and occurs at the microlevel (bedside) and macrolevel (social and policy).

INTRODUCTION

Advocacy can be defined as "the act of pleading or supporting"[1]; to advocate is to "plead in favor of."[1] Nurse advocacy may be thought of as "speaking out and speaking for patients."[2] But how does advocacy occur in nursing practice? How does an individual nurse provide a voice on behalf of patients that is heard? This article reviews the concept of patient advocacy and the role of nurses. Challenges to advocacy activities are presented and strategies for effective advocacy practice are discussed.

Understanding Nurse Advocacy

The role of nurses as patient advocates is embraced by nursing. The International Council of Nurses[3] and the American Nurses Association[4] (ANA) include advocacy within their definitions of nursing. Additionally, through its foundational documents—*Nursing's Social Policy Statement*, *Nursing: Scope and Standards of Practice*, and *Code of Ethics for Nurses*—the ANA[4–6] identifies the professional and ethical duties of nurses to advocate for the health, safety, and rights of patients. Yet, these organizations and documents do not define the concept of advocacy and there is no consensus of meaning within the nursing literature.[2,7,8] Furthermore, the discussion of patient advocacy in the literature has been criticized as philosophic and lacking

[a] St. David's School of Nursing, Texas State University, 1555 University Blvd., Round Rock, TX 78665, USA; [b] School of Nursing, University of Texas at Austin, 1710 Red River Street, Austin, TX 78701, USA
* Corresponding author.
E-mail address: cindyzoln@yahoo.com

Perioperative Nursing Clinics 7 (2012) 379–387
http://dx.doi.org/10.1016/j.cpen.2012.08.009
1556-7931/12/$ see front matter Published by Elsevier Inc.
periopnursing.theclinics.com

empiric research.[8–10] How is advocacy translated into practice when it is not understood?

Several studies have explored nurses' experiences to expound an understanding of patient advocacy. Nurses describe patient advocacy behaviors as teaching, informing, and supporting[11]; educating, communicating with the health care team, questioning, and ensuring adequate care[9]; analyzing, counseling, responding, shielding, and whistle-blowing activities—and advocacy is expressed as "voicing responsiveness."[8] These behaviors describe a process occurring within a nurse's relationship with a patient.

Advocacy may be considered a process that includes specific behaviors characterized by "safeguarding patients' autonomy, acting on behalf of patients, and championing social justice in the provision of health care."[7(p106)] Advocacy is not limited to the microlevel (bedside) but also occurs at the macrolevel (community and social). Additionally, advocacy behaviors are context based—"nurses may take different actions to advocate for patients in different clinical situations."[12(p64)] For instance, a nurse may act to safeguard an individual patient yet take no action to affect the circumstances (eg, policy), contributing to the occurrence of the particular situation.

Vaartio and colleagues[8] found that, although advocacy was experienced as a universal right of patients and a duty of nurses, "not all nurses wanted to advocate."[(p290)] Nurse-patient relationship factors (eg, interpersonal dialogue and contextual sensitivity) were important factors in the advocacy process. The importance of the nurse-patient relationship to advocacy is a consistent finding in the literature. Interest in a patient's experience strengthened the advocacy efforts.[8] To advocate effectively, nurses need to understand what is in a patient's best interest in a particular situation and what actions best safeguard that patient.[7] Understanding of the organizational environment is important to implement advocacy actions effectively.

Interpersonal relatedness occurring within the nurse-patient relationship has been identified as central to the advocacy process.[11] Advocacy behaviors include interventions both for and with patients and involve interactions among the nurse-patient, patient-environment, nurse-environment, and nurse-patient-environment contexts.[11] Although Shirley[13] considers advocacy "focused on the achievement of patient autonomy,"[(p18)] she cautions against focusing too narrowly on an individual and argues that patients are embedded in families and communities and cannot be "autonomous" as isolated individuals; this relationality is an important ethical aspect of practice.

MacDonald[14] analyzed themes from qualitative studies exploring nurses' advocacy experiences to clarify the concept of advocacy in nursing practice. The significance of the nurse-patient relationship and the importance of knowing the patient were identified as substantial themes. Relational ethics, which emphasizes the experience of relationships in influencing moral choices, is offered as a philosophy to enhance understanding of how nurses make advocacy choices.[14] The quality of nurses' relationships with all individuals in the work environment becomes important from an ethical perspective: "The workplace culture in health care institutions has a profound impact on the moral agency of nurses."[14(p125)]

Although nurses' often consider patient advocacy within the context of supporting individual patients, a broader context that includes the organization and community is proposed. Shirley[13] discusses advocacy in the context of social justice—when a nurse may need to address an individual's expressed wishes (autonomy) while managing overall resources to "ensure care for those who need it most."[(p23)] Bu and Jezewski[7] identify advocacy at the macrosocial level and suggest that nurses should change policies that interfere with patients' health care as well as "championing social justice in the provision of health care." Paquin[15] refers to social justice advocacy as an "upstream" approach, which focuses on underlying systemic problems and enables lasting solutions.

Importance of Nursing's Voice

Nurses have a unique perspective. Because of their close proximity and continuity with patients, nurses have the opportunity to come to know patients, to establish a therapeutic relationship, and to serve as an interface for patients and the rest of the health care team. Nurses are also at the sharp end of potential errors—often the last opportunity to prevent an error from actually occurring. Nurses provide a protective role for patients and organizations through patient advocacy efforts. By raising concerns about individual or organizational issues (eg, staffing, questionable clinical practices, and systems breakdowns), organizations are able to respond to resolve issues potentially affecting patient safety.

Some authors challenge nurses' role as patient advocates, arguing that nurses lack sufficient autonomy and power to advocate effectively, especially in regard to systemic concerns.[10,16,17] Collective advocacy, for example, through professional organizations, is offered as a more powerful strategy that serves society as a whole and avoids personal consequences to nurses.[16,17]

Individual consequences to nurses who advocate can be severe: in 2009, 2 nurses from Winkler County, Texas, were charged with a third-degree felony for reporting a physician to the Texas Medical Board (**Box 1**).[18] There are several other instances of retaliation for patient advocacy efforts reported in the literature.[18–20] McDonald and Ahern[21] examined the professional consequences to nurses who reported incompetent, unethical, or illegal situations to someone in a position to correct the situation. Official reprisals (reprimand, demotion, suspension, and referral to a psychiatrist) were experienced by 28% of the participants (N = 63) and unofficial reprisals (threats, ostracism, and pressure to resign) were experienced by all the participants.

The cost of speaking up can be great for an individual nurse who advocates for patients. But what are the costs of silence? *Silence Kills: The Seven Crucial Conversations in Healthcare*[22] indicates that when health care workers do not raise crucial issues, patient outcomes are negatively affected. Since the Institute of Medicine published its landmark report, *To Err is Human: Building a Safer Health System*,[23] revealing that medical errors kill approximately 100,000 people in US hospitals each year, organizations have been urged to create cultures of safety that better protect patients from

---

Box 1
Winkler County whistle-blowers

In 2009, 2 long-term employees of Winkler County Memorial Hospital, a 20-bed critical access hospital in rural west Texas, were fired from their jobs and charged with a third-degree felony for misuse of official information. Their offense? They anonymously reported a physician to the Texas Medical Board for concerns that his practice did not meet standards of care.

When their internal reports were stifled by the hospital administrator, Anne Mitchell and Vickilyn Galle believed they had no choice but to report externally to prevent further patient harm. The physician elicited the assistance of the county sheriff, and later prosecuting attorney, to identify the complainants and attempt to silence them.

With the assistance of a legal defense fund established by the Texas Nurses Association (TNA) and supported by nurses, physicians, attorneys, and others across the country, the nurses successfully defended their right to advocate for patient safety.

(see www.texasnurses.org for a full historical account).

harm. A critical component of a safe culture is communication: "An environment exists where an individual staff member, no matter what his or her job description, has the right and the responsibility to speak up on behalf of a patient."[24(p157)] Organizations committed to a culture of safety should invite staff to speak out about concerns.

A culture supporting open communication is critical to support nurse advocacy efforts and patient safety. The 2 most important reasons nurses identify for not report-ing a concern are fear of retaliation and belief that nothing will be done.[25,26] The act of raising concerns is considered high risk and low benefit.[26] The conflict nurses expe-rience between their professional duty to raise concerns and their fear of negative repercussions results in moral distress.[27] Often there is little support for nurses expe-riencing moral distress. Although nurses experiencing bioethical dilemmas in practice are generally able to seek the consult of an organizational ethics committee, such a support system rarely exists for issues related to organizational ethics.

Ray[20] proposes a relational ethics approach to establishing an organizational infra-structure for the development of a moral community. A moral community creates "moral space"[(p441)] for ethical concerns to be brought forward and considered in a context of mutual respect and engagement: "A relational ethics approach could eliminate the negative consequences of internal whistleblowing by fostering an inter-dependent moral community to address ethical concerns."[(p444)]

There is a role and need for collective advocacy, particularly in the policy realm, and this occurs most effectively through professional organizations. Unreported problems at the organization level, however, are lost opportunities to prevent harm and improve patient safety. Strategies to improve the effectiveness of nurse advocacy activities need to occur at all levels to maximize positive effects on patient care and outcomes.

Strategies for Effective Advocacy

Individual nurses

Nurses own an individual and collective role in improving the effectiveness of patient advocacy and promoting patient safety. As individuals, nurses may lack knowledge about their professional duty, legal protections, organizational policies and proce-dures, and support within the organizational structure (eg, ethics, performance improvement, staffing, or shared governance committees). Additionally, nurses may lack skill in articulating their concerns in a manner that invites problem solving. To provide a voice that is heard and responded to, individual nurses should

- Know the laws and regulations affecting their practice. This includes state nursing practice acts as well as state and federal reporting requirements and advocacy and whistle-blower protections. State boards of nursing and profes-sional nursing organizations are resources.
- Understand policies and procedures for raising concerns in their work environ-ment. Organizations typically have a structure or chain of command for reporting and responding to patient care concerns. Different kinds of issues may be referred differently (eg, concern about a physician may go to amedical director, staffing concern to a staffing committee, nurse competency concern to a nurse manager, and billing concern to a corporate compliance officer). Nurses who are informed about problem-solving structures within the organization are best able to make their voice heard.
- Contribute to a positive practice environment in the organization. Most organiza-tions offer opportunities for nurses to participate in performance improvement efforts, whether through active committee involvement (eg, hospital-acquired pressure ulcer reduction task force, staffing committee, or performance

improvement council) or through less formal activities, such as staff meetings, surveys, or focus groups. Nurses have knowledge about ways to improve their work but, unless shared constructively, that knowledge is useless.

- Improve their communication skills to provide a voice that can be heard. A passionate complaint, for instance, "This assignment is unsafe!" leaves a supervisor in a poor position to respond. By specifically articulating, however, the nature of a concern—"The way the surgeries are scheduled, my circulating assignments will overlap 2 cases. Safe practice requires me to cover 1 case at a time. Can we relook at the assignment?"—a supervisor understands precisely the nature of the concern and potential solution.
- Join and become involved in professional organizations. Nurses are more able to be influential in policy changes that support patient safety through nurse advocacy collectively than individually. Unfortunately, only a small minority of nurses belong to any professional organization.

Organizations

As MacDonald[14] stated, the organizational culture exerts a "profound impact" on the moral agency of nurses. It is up to the organization and the nurse leaders within them to create cultures of safety in which all voices are encouraged without the threat of retaliation. Managers, specifically, are integral in creating an open culture for communication where nurses believe they can speak up and be heard.[28] Nurse leaders should

- Educate nursing staff about laws, regulations, and accreditation standards and how established policies and procedures implement these requirements.
- Ensure that nurses understand the chain of command within the organization for various patient care concerns and coach staff in articulating their concerns using established channels.
- Reinforce a culture of safety by encouraging staff to raise concerns. Be clear that retaliation is not tolerated and take action if negative repercussions are experienced.
- Be responsive! Along with fear of retaliation, concern that no action will be taken as a result of raising concerns is among the top 2 reasons why nurses did not make reports. Ensure that a feedback process exists so that nurses who raise concerns know their concerns are taken seriously. Although full disclosure of action taken may not be possible, a nurse raising a concern should know that the problem was investigated and that an appropriate response resulted.
- Create opportunities for nurses to be involved in improvement activities. *The Future of Nursing: Leading Change, Advancing Health*[29] describes the imperative that every nurse be a leader in innovation to change care systems and raise the bar on patient outcomes. Nurse leaders should create the space within the organization for such innovation to occur.

Professional associations

As discussed by several investigators, advocacy at the macrolevel is most effectively achieved through professional associations.[16,17] Professional associations can promote policy change that supports individual advocacy efforts across the profession. Several examples of advocacy at the macrolevel by the TNA are discussed.

The nurse advocate certificate program A unique program by the TNA introduced the role of a nurse advocate who supports nurses in their efforts to speak out on patient safety and quality-of-care concerns. The Nurse Advocate Certificate Program (NACP) prepared hospital-based experts in internal mechanisms for raising and resolving patient care concerns (eg, policies and procedures and chain of command), external reporting avenues, and processes for maximizing legal protections when engaging in patient advocacy activities. The concept of the nurse advocate is consistent with relational ethics and cultures of safety. A nurse advocate also provides nurses at risk of moral distress with a resource to resolve ethical concerns.

The NACP included a 2-day workshop covering the role of nurses as patient advocates, organizational characteristics of a culture of safety, whistle-blower and advocacy laws and regulations, conflict resolution, and organizational policy considerations. Participants received a resource handbook and consultation and support from TNA program directors. After completing the training workshop, nurse advocates work within their hospitals' structure to develop and implement the advocate role. Program participants are eligible to take an examination to certify their expertise as nurse advocates. Approximately 35 nurses completed the NACP. Sponsoring hospitals included urban medical centers, midsized community hospitals, and a rural critical access hospital of 32 beds. Participants identified the need to educate leadership in the organization as a first step in implementing the nurse advocate role.[30]

Texas Hospital Safe Staffing Law (2009) Since nurse staffing regulations were implemented in Texas in 2002, research substantiating the relationship between nurse staffing and patient outcomes has flourished (**Box 2**). In 2007, the TNA established a nursing task force to evaluate implementation of existing staffing regulations, consider best practices in nurse staffing, and make recommendations to the organization. Recommendations were adopted by 2008 TNA House of Delegates via a resolution directing TNA to continue its support of direct care nurses in staffing decisions, explore ways to strengthen existing staffing regulations, and investigate strategies to evaluate compliance and effectiveness of staffing requirements. These directives were pursued by TNA's Governmental Affairs Committee, who collaborated with the Texas Hospital Association, Texas Organization of Nurse Executives, and the Texas Nursing

---

Box 2
Hospital Safe Staffing Law (2009)

Important provisions of the Texas Hospital Safe Staffing Law directly affecting nursing's voice included

- The staffing committee must consist of 60% direct care nurses, selected by their peers and representing all clinical areas of the hospital where nursing is practiced. The chief nursing officer must sit on the committee and the committee must report directly to the hospital board.

- The nurse staffing committee is responsible for soliciting, reviewing, assessing, and responding to staffing concerns. Retaliation against a nurse reporting staffing concerns is illegal.

- The nurse staffing plan must be used to guide nursing assignments. Variances in actual and desired staffing are reported to the nurse staffing committee.

- The nurse staffing committee evaluates the effectiveness of the staffing plan considering nurse-sensitive patient outcome measures (selected by the committee) and variances in actual and desired staffing. This evaluation is reported semiannually to the hospital board.

- The hospital must make the staffing plan and current staffing levels available to nurses every shift. The hospital must also report staffing information to the Texas Department of State Health Services (TDSHS) as part of its annual survey process.

Mandatory overtime is prohibited.[31]

Legislative Agenda Coalition to develop legislation. In 2009 the Hospital Safe Staffing Law was passed by the 81st Texas Legislature. The new law built on existing regulations requiring hospital staffing committees and enhanced nursing's influence and hospital accountability for adequate staffing.

The Hospital Safe Staffing Law renewed and strengthened nursing's voice in staffing—a major concern of hospital nurses and a critical factor in patient outcomes. The law purposely requires the voice of direct care nurses in developing, evaluating, and reporting nurse staffing. Further, the 2 primary concerns of nurses—fear that nothing will be done and fear of negative repercussions—are directly addressed. The Hospital Safe Staffing Law was passed by nurses working collectively and collaboratively with key stakeholders and could not have been accomplished by an individual effort.

The Patient Advocacy Protections Law (2011) Nurses understand never events to be adverse occurrences that are unambiguous, serious, and preventable[32]; they should never happen. The grievous retaliation that occurred against 2 nurses in Winkler County, Texas, who filed a good faith report to the Texas Medical Board about patient safety concerns[18] constituted a never event. When a never event occurs in health care, immediate and intense action occurs to minimize recurrence. Decisive action in response to the Winkler County event encompassed the Patient Advocacy Protections Law (PAPL) initiated by the TNA in the 82nd Texas Legislature.

Texas nurses enjoy some of the strongest patient advocacy protections in the country, yet the possibility of criminal charges for patient advocacy activities was never anticipated. Passage of the PAPL helps ensure that what occurred to Mitchell and Vickilyn Galle in Winkler County never happens again. Specifically, the law

- Establishes "good faith" rather than "without malice" as the standard for making protected reports (The prosecutor based much of his case against Mitchell on the supposition that she did not like the physician she reported rather than on her belief that his practice was unsafe.)
- Provides immunity from criminal liability
- Protects
  - Nurses who advise nurses about their rights
  - Nurses from all persons in a position to retaliate (not just the employer)
  - The nurse advocate role

No law can guarantee retaliation will never occur, but laws can establish conditions that strongly discourage behavior and provide remedies to nurses if they are retaliated against. The TNA reported Winkler County Hospital to the TDSHS for illegal retaliation against Mitchell and Galle. After its investigation, TDSHS agreed and fined the hospital the maximum allowed for the offense: $650 per nurse—an insignificant penalty unlikely to deter recurrence. Similarly, after investigating the reported physician, the Texas Medical Board determined that, in additional to several patient care violations, the physician had illegally retaliated against the nurses. The Board levied the maximum fine allowed for the offense: $5000. The PAPL enhances potential penalties for retaliation by authorizing agencies to impose fines significant enough to act as a deterrent (up to $25,000).[33]

Professional associations play an important role in supporting advocacy efforts by nurses by establishing social policies that protect patients as well as their advocates. Perhaps nurses' duty to advocate individually for the health, safety, and rights of patients should be extended as a duty to act collectively through professional associations as well as individually.

SUMMARY

At the 2011 National Nursing Ethics Conference, held in Los Angeles, Ann Hamric, PhD, RN, FAAN, stated in a question-and-answer session after her plenary presentation, "It should never be an act of moral courage for a nurse to advocate for a patient."[34] When Winkler County nurses Anne Mitchell and Vickilyn Galle prepared to testify to the Senate Committee on Health and Human Services in support of the PAPL, they commented that they had not done anything special: "we just did what any nurse would do for her patients" (Anne Mitchell, PhD, RN, FAAN, personal communication, 2011). The unfortunate reality is that negative repercussions for patient advocacy are real; too often moral courage is necessary to speak up, and not all nurses are able to effectively advocate for their patients.

Patient advocacy has many paths, including supporting patient autonomy and decision making, reporting patient care concerns, refusing to engage in behavior that violates a duty to a patient, participating in decisions about nursing practice, and changing health care policy. The public depends on such patient advocacy efforts to ensure that care achieves safety and quality standards. Retaliation for patient advocacy efforts has a chilling effect on potential advocates. No one benefits when nurses are silenced. Nurses at all levels of practice have a role and a duty to move beyond rhetoric and support patient advocacy.

REFERENCES

1. Dictionary.com: advocacy. Available at: http://dictionary.reference.com/browse/advocacy?s=t&ld=1031. Accessed June 8, 2012.
2. Hanks RG. The lived experience of nursing advocacy. Nurs Ethics 2008;15(4): 468–77.
3. International Council of Nurses (2010). Definition of nursing. Available at: http://www.icn.ch/about-icn/icn-definition-of-nursing/. Accessed June 15, 2012.
4. American Nurses Association. Nursing's social policy statement: the essence of the profession. Author: Silver Spring (MD): 2010.
5. American Nurses Association. Nursing: scope and standards of practice. Author: Silver Spring (MD): 2010.
6. American Nurses Association. Code of ethics for nurses with interpretive statements. Author: Silver Spring (MD): 2001.
7. Bu X, Jezewski MA. Developing a mid-range theory of patient advocacy through concept analysis. J Adv Nurs 2006;57(1):101–10.
8. Vaartio H, Leino-Kilpi H, Salanterä S, et al. Nursing advocacy: how is it defined by patients and nurses, what does it involve and how is it experienced? Scand J Caring Sci 2006;20:282–92.
9. Hanks RG. The medical-surgical nurse perspective of the advocate role. Nurs Forum 2010;45(2):97–107.
10. Hewitt J. A critical review of the arguments debating the role of the nurse. J Adv Nurs 2002;37(5):439–45.
11. Chafey K, Rhea M, Shannon AM, et al. Characterizations of advocacy by practicing nurses. J Prof Nurs 1998;14(1):43–52.
12. Bu X, Wu YB. Development and psychometric evaluation of the instrument: attitude toward patient advocacy. Res Nurs Health 2007;31:63–75.
13. Shirley JL. Limits of autonomy in nursing's moral discourse. Adv Nurs Sci 2007; 30(1):14–25.
14. MacDonald H. Relational ethics and advocacy in nursing: literature review. J Adv Nurs 2007;57(2):119–26.

15. Paquin SO. Social justice advocacy in nursing: what is it? How do we get there? Creative Nursing 2011;17(2):63–7.
16. Mahlin M. Individual patient advocacy, collective responsibility and activism within professional nursing associations. Nursing Ethics 2010;17(2):247–54.
17. Welchman J, Griener GG. Patient advocacy and professional associations: individual and collective responsibilities. Nursing Ethics 2005;12(3):296–303.
18. Texas Nurses Association (no date). Advocacy: Winkler County Nurse Whistleblower History. Retrieved on 6/17/12 from http://www.texasnurses.org/displaycommon.cfm?an=1&subarticlenbr=597.
19. Texas Nurses Association. Another whistleblower victory. Texas Nursing 2000;1–2 August.
20. Ray SL. Whistleblowing and organizational ethics. Nursing Ethics 2006;13(4):438–45.
21. McDonald S, Ahern K. The professional consequences of whistleblowing by nurses. Journal of Professional Nursing 2000;16(6):313–21.
22. Maxfield D, Grenny J, McMillan R, et al. Silence kills: the seven crucial conversations in healthcare. Executive Summary. VitalSmarts™ Industry Watch 2005.
23. Kohn LT, Corrigan JM, Donaldson MS. To Err is Human: Building a safer health system. Washington, D. C.: National Academies Press; 2000.
24. Sammer CE, Lykens K, Singh KP, et al. What is patient safety culture? A review of the literature. Journal of Nursing Scholarship 2010;42(2):156–65.
25. Black LM. Tragedy into policy: a quantitative study of nurses' attitudes toward patient advocacy activities. American Journal of Nursing 2011;111(6):26–35.
26. Attree M. Factors influencing nurses' decisions to raise concerns about care quality. Journal of Nursing Management 2007;15:392–402.
27. Corley MC. Nurse moral distress: a proposed theory and research agenda. Nursing Ethics 2002;9(6):636–50.
28. Garon M. Speaking up, being heard: registered nurses' perceptions of workplace communication. Journal of Nursing Management 2012;20:361–71.
29. Institute of Medicine. The Future of Nursing: Leading Change, Advancing Health. Washington, D. C.: The National Academies Press; 2011.
30. Zolnierek C, Willmann J. Texas Nurses Association's Nurse Advocate Certificate Program: Supporting Patient Advocacy Activities by Nurses. Poster session presented at the National Nursing Et. Los Angeles, 2011. Available at: http://dictionary.reference.com/browse/advocacyhicsConference.
31. Zolnierek C. In setting safe staffing levels, nurses know best. Texas Nursing Voice 2009;3(3):5–8.
32. Agency for Healthcare Research and Quality. Patient safety primers: never event. 2006. Available at: http://psnet.ahrq.gov/primer.aspx?primerID=3. Accessed June 17, 2012.
33. Zolnierek C. Testimony presented to the Texas Senate Committee on Health and Human Services on Senate Bill 192 (82R) Patient Advocacy Protections Bill. March 1, 2011.
34. Hamric AB. The price of advocacy: dealing with moral distress. Plenary presentation at the 2011 National Nursing Ethics Conference. Los Angeles, March. 2011.

On Advocating as a Nurse

Kathryn M. Tart, EdD, MSN, BA

KEYWORDS

• Advocacy • Decision-making • Influence

KEY POINTS

- In nursing, there are 6 levels of advocacy for health care needs, patients, and the profession itself.
- This article describes the process that enables nurses to establish themselves as influential advocates.

Advocacy is one of the professional nursing roles. Nurses feel comfortable in this role when it comes to advocating for the patient at the bedside and know they make a difference for patients who cannot speak for themselves. Nurses can be staunchly loyal in their patient advocacy as they assist patients in health outcomes. Yet, they can also advocate for their patients on a larger scale in these same purposeful ways. Each individual nurse can contribute in purposeful ways that make a difference for patients and assist in health outcomes. Ultimately, the nurse can become comfortable in the role of nurse advocate whether at the bedside or in an environment away from the bedside.

Nurses may ask themselves, "As a nurse advocate, how do I make a difference? What are my first steps? How do I deal with the political climate of the times?" A nurse advocate can make a list of the items, ideas, values, concepts or thoughts that make a difference to patients, the nursing profession, and health care. Organizing thoughts can be a good first step to articulating professional values in advocating for patients and nursing issues. Ultimately, the nurse will communicate nursing issues at a state and national level that impact the practice and policy of nursing. The nurse will want to explore the levels of nurse advocacy in the political climate. Each of the six levels described below will take the nurse into a deeper commitment to advocacy.

The first level of advocacy is *voting*. Voting is a basic right and it is as simple as obtaining a voter's registration card. Individual nurses engage in advocating by making their voices heard through this first important level of advocacy.

The second level is *writing* a congressman or senator at the state or national level. Expressing one's position on issues in a letter or email helps the congressman or

Funding Sources: None.
Conflict of Interest: None.
School of Nursing, University of Houston Victoria, 3007 North Ben Wilson, Victoria, TX 77901, USA
E-mail address: tartk@uhv.edu

Perioperative Nursing Clinics 7 (2012) 389–391
http://dx.doi.org/10.1016/j.cpen.2012.08.005
1556-7931/12/$ – see front matter © 2012 Elsevier Inc. All rights reserved.

senator in a number of ways. First, it informs or teaches the elected official about the issue. A nurse is someone from whom the elected official wants to hear, and officials need to know how the issue affects his or her constituents. Secondly, elected official's staff tally the number of letters and emails that come in regarding the issues. One representative noted that every time she votes on an issue she reviews the number of letters and emails she received for and against the issue. The tally is important for her vote.

Next, when writing a letter or email, nurses thank the official for the service they render to the state or nation. Showing appreciation is very important and opens officials to the issue, bill or the topic to which the nurse is writing. Nurses should let the official know of their expertise and give personal stories on the impact of the issue to their constituents. Clarity in the correspondence about the response nurses seek from the official is important. Lastly, officials will need the nurse's contact information. Offering themselves as a resource for any further information or questions on the issue to which they are writing is also an important step for the nurse advocates to take.

The third level of advocacy is to *attend* a public speech, rally or meeting. When attending nurses should be aware of the nature of the event and how it relates to the issues for which they are most interested in advocating. They may hear and talk to many individuals with varying levels of opinions and may also hear the elected official's position on issues. When nurses speak or ask a question, they should identify themselves as nurses and reveal their specialty in nursing. The public recognizes nurses as experts and values the profession's knowledge, reputation, care and trust. Nursing positions establish respect and add to the base of nursing advocacy. Nurses' introductions will establish their expertise and their issue will be regarded by the listeners.

Next, the nurse must show appreciation by thanking the elected official or the meeting organizers. Nurses' speech or questions should be articulated in such a way that listeners can remember what they say or remember their question. Short statements or questions that are to the point can have a great impact. Again, nurses should ask for a response and show appreciation. Nurses also have the opportunity to model civil dialogue and behavior in public events which add to the nurses' credibility.

The fourth level of advocacy is *meeting and visiting* a congressman or senator at the *local* office. Elected officials' hard work is done at the home office where legislative agendas are crafted and bills are written. Nurses can call or email the office to make an appointment to meet with the elected official or their staff members bringing written information and data on the issue(s) the nurses wish to discuss. Nurses should bring business cards so the elected official or staff member can contact them at a future date for information or to ask questions. Arriving a little before the appointment a nurse should let the elected official or staff member know he or she is a nurse and thank them for the work they are doing.

Nurse advocates should find a way to connect with the elected official or staff member. The connection may be the official has have a relative or friend in the health care world, or the connection may be their own personal experience or encounter with health care, either positive or negative. Nurse must listen to what the elected officials or staffs tells them and make their connections from those stories. Many times nurses can weave others experiences into the issues nurses wish to discuss.

The information and data nurses bring to such a meeting is also important and should be shared. If the elected official is new nurse advocates have a perfect opportunity to teach the official or staffer about nursing and health care. Office holders are as eager to learn as they are interested in representing their new constituents. Nurse advocates should express appreciation for the official's time and offer to help: for instance, to serve on a task force or present information at other events. One question many nurses may have is, "why would the elected official listen to me? I did not vote for them, nor am

I of the same party." A nurse advocate needs to remember that the elected official represents all people in their district regardless of their party affiliation or vote. Elected officials want to win votes and will listen, as representatives, to what constituents have to say. The nurse advocate should write a letter or email of thanks for the visit and recap the intent and outcome of the visit, again providing contact information.

If the nurse meets the elected official or staff person again in the future, he or she should remind them of the health care connection that they share and ask about family members or friends. The official will immediately appreciate the nurse's personal interest in them and be open to listening. In this way nurse advocates can build relationships over time and through personal and professional connections. The elected official or staff person knows the advocate as an expert and can ask for information in the future and depend on the advocate's follow through, trust his or her expertise and seek the advocate's opinion on issues that matter to their constituents.

The fifth level of advocacy is *meeting or visiting* a congressman or senator at the *state or national* offices. If nurse advocates have met officials at the home office, the nurse advocate will certainly be remembered! There is a fondness for visitors from home, especially ones who have been met before. Officials know the nurse advocates have made a special trip to see them and the advocate's issues are very important for them to consider. Nurses should call or email for an appointment and follow the same steps as they would for a visit at home. Advocating as a nurse at this level is powerful because the elected official or staff member knows the importance of the visit and respects the issues for which the nurse is advocating. The nurse is also in the position at this point to let his or her personality come through. These relationships can help shape opportunities for future advocacy issues. Nurses must let their legislators know they are ready to step up to the plate in health care and advocacy for patients.

The last level of advocacy is to *work* for a person running for an elected position or for a political party. The work is most frequently voluntary. The candidate and the party highly value and respect the work, making the nurse very connected. The nurse can also increase connections to influential community people, corporations and other politicians.

Moreover, nurses can increase their connections and advocacy in ways that influence the community and profession. They can work on shared governance boards of their hospitals. They can serve on school boards in their communities. Nurses can serve in their professional organizations. The more connections the nurse advocate has, the more opportunity they have for professional advocacy. Supporting other health care workers professionally in the workplace and through a unified voice on large social issues can increase strength and self-esteem among nurses.[1]

A nursing student wrote in her journal: "After three days of lecture in the perioperative nursing elective, I have concluded that the most important thing I have learned is that the nurse's #1 responsibility is to be the patient advocate at all times." In a few years and as a more experienced nurse, this person should loyally hold this sentiment at the bedside and in the wider environment of the nurse's community, state and nation. What are the opportunities each nurse has to advocate for patients? What will their next steps be in nursing advocacy? Nursing is an awesome profession! We should thank each nurse for advocating for the patients he or she serves and for being smart people who care about health care and doing what is right for their patients and profession.

Thank you for being a nurse advocate!

REFERENCE

1. Des Jardin KE. Political involvement in nursing – education and empowerment. AORN J 2001;74(4):467–71, 473–9, 481–2.

Communicating with Your Legislator

Joanne D. Oliver, RN, BSN, CNOR

KEYWORDS

- Legislation • Advocacy • Health care costs • Health care environment

KEY POINTS

- Involvement in the legislative process is an effective way to influence access to health care, health care costs, and the role of nursing in the health care environment.
- Research legislation being presented, formulate a personal plan for your own involvement, get to know your legislators and communicate with them consistently.
- The 3.1 million registered nurses in the U.S. can educate and influence legislators and promote a positive future for nursing.

INTRODUCTION

The 3.1 million registered nurses in the United States comprise a large basis for exerting strong influence on the future direction of health care. Active involvement in advocating for nursing is a matter of taking the first step. For most nurses, involvement begins with an issue of personal interest or a request to contact legislators about a bill. That request usually includes "immediately!" You do not have to wait for a crisis. Developing a relationship with your legislators before you need their support puts you in a better position when you contact them about something specific. Nurses who are apathetic or indifferent allow others to make the decisions that affect our profession; sometimes those decisions are not what we would wish to have happened. Think of the influence that 3.1 million voices would have on the decision makers if every nurse participated in the process. It takes little effort to make a significant difference. This article guides nurses through the steps in developing those essential relationships and increase their comfort levels with getting involved.

A PERSONAL PERSPECTIVE

Legislators must make decisions about a large number of issues in a short time frame. They cannot be experts in every field, so they rely heavily on their staffers to research issues and on the experts in those fields with whom they have developed

Healthcare Resources, Houston, Tx 77069, USA.
E-mail address: joliver@hcresources.net

Perioperative Nursing Clinics 7 (2012) 393–396
http://dx.doi.org/10.1016/j.cpen.2012.08.013
1556-7931/12/$ – see front matter © 2012 Elsevier Inc. All rights reserved.

relationships. They value the expertise of their nurse constituents when health care issues arise. You can be your legislator's go-to nurse.

Almost 20 years ago, the author was asked by a colleague to testify before the Senate Health & Human Services Committee at the State Capitol. Having never done anything like this, she was nervous, but her passion about the issue motivated her to agree. She began to read the script her colleague had given her to read to the committee. Various senators interrupted with questions and comments, giving her an opportunity to explain to them, with examples from her practice. When they began hearing about the reality of nursing, they started to listen.

During the most recent legislative session, a congressman called the author from the floor of the House, asking for her opinion related to a bill on which he was about to vote. She is her legislators' go-to nurse, the person he relies on for information about nursing and health care. She invested some time in developing that important relationship, which has earned her the privilege of participating in decisions that affect nursing practice. No one knows more about nursing than nurses.

When you are passionate about your patients, it is easy to get involved in advocating for their safety and for the nursing profession. Most issues that affect nursing practice have an ultimate impact on patients as well. Advocacy is part of a professional nurse's dedication to the nursing profession.

DEVELOPING THAT IMPORTANT RELATIONSHIP

Although it helps to have a mentor when you first start, do not think you cannot do it on your own. Remember, no one knows what is best for nursing better than nurses. Remember, too, that each nursing voice is amplified by the voices of colleagues, increasing the volume and power of communication. There is a multitude of ways to get involved, to learn about what is happening in the public policy arena that affects nursing. One easy way is to seek out colleagues who already participate. Mention your interest to your colleagues at work or at a professional association meeting. Nurses who are interested in politics are excited about sharing their knowledge and experience with interested colleagues. You may quickly find yourself with a mentor.

First, you must find out who your legislators are. There are excellent online resources for locating the state and federal legislators who represent you. (**Box 1**) Every state legislature has a Web site where you can find your state legislators and capture their contact information. Your political party and voting choices do not matter when developing a relationship; legislators represent all of their constituents, regardless of political affiliation and voting record. You do not need to have an issue to discuss to make your first appointment. Your objective is to develop a relationship, to let your legislator know that you are a registered nurse who is interested in legislation involving health care, and that you are a health care expert willing to share your expertise.

Box 1
Online resources for locating state and federal legislators

US House of Representatives. http://www.house.gov/representatives/find/

US Senate (put your state in the "Find Your Senators" search box). http://www.senate.gov/index.htm

US Senator and Congressman by zip code: http://whoismyrepresentative.com/

Put "find your legislator" in the search engine of your browser. Every state has a Web site to help you locate your elected officials.

PREPARING FOR A VISIT TO DISCUSS AN ISSUE

When you plan a visit to your legislator to discuss a specific issue, some preparation will help to make the visit a success. Information about the legislator's special interests or accomplishments will help get the conversation started. Be prepared with the facts about your issue and be familiar with the points your opposition is making against the issue. Select 1 or 2 talking points to keep your presentation succinct and on target. Prepare a single-page fact sheet to leave with the legislator. Include a short summary of your position (why the legislator should support/not support the bill), bullet points of the most pertinent pieces of the legislation, and your contact information for follow-up questions or discussion.

Know who is in opposition to the bill and what the objections are. Be prepared to address what the legislator may have already heard from constituents who oppose your position. Be careful not to be argumentative or defensive. Legislators never want to be involved in turf wars. They look for ways to keep everyone happy. For example, a bill to remove barriers to advance practice nurses (APN) practicing to the level of their education and licensure may be opposed by physicians who see the bill as an encroachment on their practice. The legislator's constituents include both APNs and physicians; it is sometimes politically unwise for the legislator to take sides. Remain objective and present the facts: how many more citizens will have access to health care; how much money will be saved by providing preventive care in underserved areas and avoiding acute care costs, and so forth. The more compelling the argument that your position is in the public's best interest, the more likely the legislator is to be supportive.

When you make the appointment, let the office know the issue you would like to discuss. If legislators are not available, they will be able to schedule a meeting with the staff person responsible for researching that issue. It is valuable to develop a relationship with the staff person responsible for health care or for the bill that you are addressing. Legislators have many bills to manage, so they rely heavily on the staff person to provide the information and perspective needed to make voting decisions. Your goal is to become a trusted source of information.

HOW TO GET YOUR POINT ACROSS

When you speak with the legislator or staff person, identify the issue by bill number and the legislator(s) who introduced it. Ask whether they are familiar with the issue. You are presenting yourself to your legislator as an expert; it is essential that you know as much about the issue as possible. Identify the stakeholders who will be affected by the bill and how they will be affected. Legislators are interested in the impact of a bill on their constituents and on the bill's fiscal note: what it will cost if the bill is passed. A bill that can save money will capture a legislator's attention.

Deliver your prepared presentation. Use pictures, facts and figures, and graphs wherever possible. Bring the issue to life by describing how it affects your practice and your patients. Legislators are interested in how an issue affects their constituents. Give an example or tell a story. Personal accounts will help legislators remember you and the issue by providing a frame of reference. When you are through, be quiet and listen carefully to the legislator's questions and comments.

At the end of the meeting, thank the legislators for their time and offer to be available for further discussion, to provide any information they may have requested, and to serve as a resource on any other health care matters. Find out what form of communication is preferred; some prefer phone calls, others e-mail or written communication. Do not forget to ask, "Can I count on your support for [Bill #]?" or "Can I count on your vote against [Bill #]?" Be sure you have left a business card in addition to the fact sheet with your contact information.

HOW TO FOLLOW UP

First, write a note thanking the legislator or staff person for their time. When additional information to support your position is available, be sure that you get that into your legislator's hands. Be positive and factual in all communication; complainers are not appreciated. Whether a bill passes or fails, always send a note thanking them for their service. This is a good investment in your relationship with your legislators going forward.

PARTICIPATE ON AN ONGOING BASIS

Keep abreast of the political agendas in which you are interested. For instance, AORN legislative priorities reflect the primary interests of the specialty of perioperative nursing. Join the grassroots legislative movement of your specialty organization to keep abreast of legislative initiatives. Take action on legislative alerts; e-mails that ask you to contact your legislator (usually immediately) regarding a specific issue. The alerts usually contain the key points in a preformatted communication that you can send right away, either as it is presented or modified to reflect your relationship with the legislator. The more communication legislators receive from constituents, the more likely they are to take action on an issue.

Most states have a Nurse Day at the Capitol or a Lobby Day organized by the state nurses association. Nurses from all over the state congregate at the state capital on a specific day to visit with legislators about predefined issues affecting nursing and health care. A large group of constituents is impressive and legislators are likely to take notice.

SUMMARY

Nurses must actively participate in influencing the future of health care and the nursing profession. Involvement in the legislative process is an effective way to influence access to health care, health care costs, and the role of nursing in the health care environment. Read and research the legislation being presented, formulate a personal plan for your own involvement. Know your legislators and communicate with them consistently. Be well prepared, listen carefully, speak clearly, and be persistent. As informed, committed, and enthusiastic supporters of legislation that furthers our objectives, and opponents of legislation that interferes with our objectives, 3.1 million registered nurses can educate and influence legislators and promote the future in which we believe.

SUGGESTED READINGS

AARP issue brief: nursing shortage. AARP; 2010.

National Alliance on Mental Issues (NAMI). Advocacy Action Center. 2012.

Oliver J. Perioperative nursing and politics: where do you start? Perioperative Nursing Clinics 2009;4(1):13–5.

TCEA.org/Advocacy Resources. Tips on talking to your legislator in person. Resource Guides and Toolkits.

Texas Nurses Association. Advocacy Center. 2012.

United States Department of Labor. Bureau of Labor Statistics. Overview of Bureau of Labor Statistics on employment. 2012. Available at: http://www.bls.gov/bls/employment.htm. Accessed October 2012.

Advocating for Nurses and Patients

Creating and Maintaining a Just Culture of Safety and Advocacy in Perioperative Services

Mike Thomas, RN, MA, BSN, CNOR, MLSSBB

KEYWORDS

- Safety • Advocacy • Nursing culture

KEY POINTS

- A culture of safety and advocacy is the most effective environment in which to address workplace challenges successfully and deliver outstanding, safe patient care.
- A safe or just culture encourages employees to be vigilant, to identify and examine close calls to prevent errors.
- Such a culture emphasizes patient safety, retains employees, curbs spiraling healthcare costs, and meets regulatory and patient expectations of care.

BACKGROUND

Current work environment emphasizes continuous performance improvement, reimbursement issues, spiraling health care costs, and core measure baselines for delivering improved, evidence-based care. These driving forces are compelling a change within the health care system. A shortage of registered nurses, and an aging perioperative workforce of registered nurse, in particular, is prevalent. Organizational change is a challenge for organizations both large and small. However, a culture of safety and advocacy is the most effective environment to deliver outstanding, safe patient care, successfully address workplace challenges, and recruit and retain competent caregivers.

As we have advocated for our patients, safety issues have been managed primarily through incident- or occurrence-reporting systems and processes. This approach focuses on incidents that have already happened. A more recent approach focuses on prevention: the identification and exploration of near misses. This term is misleading; such instances are really near hits or close calls. In reality, close calls are underreported, because the transition from the shame and blame environment, in which people are punished for their mistakes, to the culture of advocacy and safety (also known as a just culture), in which errors and close calls serve as opportunities for improvement, has not been effectively made.

Surgical Services, Baylor Regional Medical Center, 4700 Alliance Blvd., Plano, TX 75093, USA
E-mail address: mike.thomas@baylorhealth.edu

Perioperative Nursing Clinics 7 (2012) 397–400
http://dx.doi.org/10.1016/j.cpen.2012.09.001
1556-7931/12/$ – see front matter © 2012 Published by Elsevier Inc.
periopnursing.theclinics.com

At present, a much keener awareness that systems and processes significantly affect the incidence of errors and close calls, and that punishing individuals does not have a significant impact on reducing medical errors is present. A process is designed to produce an outcome. When the outcome differs from what is anticipated, it is most likely the process, not the practitioner that needs fixing. A commitment to improved systems engineering does not imply that individuals don't make mistakes. The difference in a culture of advocacy and safety is that errors and near misses are approached with an open mind, a focused intention to identify the cause, and to make improvements to avoid recurrences. Individuals are encouraged to report errors and close calls that promote investigation, improvement, and prevent recurrences. Such a culture must be supported at all levels of an organization, beginning at the top.

A surgical services Director known for his commitment to safety and advocacy was given responsibility for a recently-purchased surgery center. In a very short time, the Director identified culture issues in the new center. The physical environment was inefficient, clinical practices did not meet standards, and the staff was neither engaged nor interested in learning. The Director knew that, without significant improvement, the center could not serve patients or the community well. In establishing a culture of safety and advocacy, the Director focused everyone's attention on delivering safe and effective care. The Director described the components of a culture of safety and advocacy. The staff responded when their observations were heard and appreciated, and the Director supported when they faced a challenging situation. The staff developed the confidence to address behaviors that interfered with productivity, such as bullying or refusing to explore alternatives to "the way we've always done it". Staff and surgeons learned that the culture of the center included collaborative practice. Nurses and surgeons who had bullied the team were counseled, and there was a steady progress toward evidence-based, cost-effective, collegial practice. Leaders emerged among the staff whose influence on their colleagues resulted in a more cohesive staff and a general willingness to grow professionally.

In every environment, surgical team members who continue to interfere with smooth and efficient practice and those who are hostile, who bully, or who think the rules do not apply to them are present. When the culture of safety does not "start at the top", administrators can often be persuaded to side with physicians and surgeons, anesthesia providers, and even prominent nursing staff on circumstances that they have been involved in that produced a hostile work environment. When administrators focus on profitability, increasing the bottom line to provide funding for growing modalities of care, and do not understand the impact that a culture of safety has on achieving those goals, the facility as a whole is affected. Culture begins at the top, and a culture of safety and advocacy cannot succeed if counterproductive behavior is supported and rewarded by the administration.

LEADERSHIP, ADMINISTRATIVE, AND MANAGERIAL SUPPORT

Although a culture of safety and advocacy is supported by senior leaders and management in the workplace, it is driven by the staff members. Empowerment evolves as the staff members experience support from the management and administration, and witness consistent application of standards, bylaws, and policy, with an emphasis on best practice. This approach resets expectations and provides the environment for staff members to define the change and take ownership of the process. Once the staff members trust that they will be supported, not blamed, for bringing attention to opportunities for improvement, they report errors, close calls, and unacceptable practice, including disruptive behaviors that interfere with positive outcomes.

Staff members, similar to all learners, respect teachers who walk their talk. A leader must demonstrate a willingness to practice what he preaches. One key behavior of leadership in the process of changing a culture is that the leader can never ask or demand the staff members to do anything that the leader cannot or will not do. Change without personal investment is not sustainable. As a leader demonstrates personal involvement, he or she also must clarify that supporting a culture of safety and advocacy is a condition of employment for all staff members.

Another practical reminder for managers is that "doers do what checkers check". The adage reminds us that people do what they are acknowledged and rewarded for doing. Another good reminder is that it takes 21 days to form a habit, and 21 days to break. If managers are not consistently involved in reinforcing a change in behavior for at least that period of time, the change will not be sustainable. The behaviors that a leader desires from the staff members are the ones that he or he must be role modeling, recognizing, and rewarding.

Although administration and management establish the practice culture, the staff members are the driving force for patient safety. Staff members reset the bar by expressing their concerns, ideas, and needs for resources to improve the delivery of patient care. Leaders focus on the "what" and the "why" of health care practice; staff must be empowered to develop the "how". Another key communication tool is evidence. Nurses, surgeons, and anesthesia providers are responsive to data. Any changes recommended must be supported with evidence, so that providers can relate to the impact a change will have on patient care and professional practice.

MOVING FROM THE PRESENT INTO THE FUTURE

Change is an evolutionary process; it does not happen overnight. Implementing a culture of safety and advocacy occurs as leaders begin to demonstrate their support for the culture and staff members begin to develop respect and trust. New behaviors develop slowly, and the process follows the steps of the nursing process: ADPIE (assess, diagnosis, plan, implement, and evaluate). First steps include an assessment of the current state of the organization. Getting from here to there requires an understanding of the elements that support the here, the current situation. Preparation for a change should include a review of bylaws, policy, procedure, and resources. A good understanding of the underlying structure and the processes that make the organization function the way it does is necessary to plan for effective improvement and change. The current status establishes a baseline against which progress can be measured.

A certain degree of inertia is associated with any culture within an organization. Change is a slow process. Humans are most likely to repeat familiar behaviors, especially if they have been positively reinforced. Good planning and significant effort is essential or inertia will pull an organization back into familiar routines. Identifying behaviors that need to change and exploring ways to reinforce new behaviors are essential steps in overcoming the organization's inertia and progressing toward the goal. Consistency in expectations and responses to behavior is critical. Administrative and leadership support is essential. Transparency encourages respect and trust, and promotes the understanding of the rationale for change and a clear picture of expectations.

When incidents or close calls are reviewed in private or by peer review committees, staff should know that the incident is receiving full attention, even when they are not privy to the specifics of the incident or the outcome of an investigation.

Although change itself is a slow process, all facets of the change process must occur simultaneously, effectively shocking the system and overcoming the initial defensiveness and cultural inertia. Simultaneous implementation brings everyone on board at

---

Speak so that others Will Hear

In the doctors' lounge, a physician was expressing, rather heatedly, his disdain for the Surgical Care Improvement Program measures. A colleague interrupted to say, "This isn't about the government telling you how to practice medicine; it's about the government telling you how they will reimburse you. Your outcomes determine how you will be paid. The practices they require are based on evidence that will produce the outcomes they want. Outcomes determine how we get paid." The physician replied that he had not looked at it that way.

Refocusing a topic from an emotional perspective to a meaningful position supported by evidence quickly quelled the diversion and got the meeting back on track. If an individual can be made to understand the positive outcomes of a situation, he or she is more like to comply with a request for a change in practice.

---

one time. Addressing complainers and resistors is easy when the goals, process, and expectations have been clearly defined, and when most of their colleagues are moving forward with the program.

Triangular Approach to Nursing Evidence-Based Practice Toward Improvement
A Starter Kit to Assess Research Strength and Enhance Patient Outcomes

Patti S. Grant, RN, BSN, MS, CIC

KEYWORDS

- Nursing evidence-based practice • Self-paced nursing EBP starter kit
- Patient safety • Culture of safety • Triangular approach to nursing EBP

KEY POINTS

- Nursing evidence-based practice (EBP) starter kit for smaller health care facilities.
- Novel triangular approach to nursing EBP to consider strength of evidence, time management, and a culture of safety.
- Internet-based references suggested for novel EBP triangular approach.
- Suggested safety dialogue and references for nurse empowerment toward furthering safety culture.
- Application of Stephen R. Covey's "7 Habits" Circle of Influence and Time Management Matrix toward implementation of nursing EBP.

This issue of *Perioperative Clinics* is focused on nurse advocacy and includes various dynamics involved with keeping the patient safe through the power of nurse-driven actions. A major component of this quest includes the content expertise of this issue's authors related to specific populations. That being said, a query for "evidence-based practice" (EBP) in PubMed[1] produces more than 68,000 articles, so how does an author focus on EBP to promote nurse advocacy without reinventing the wheel?

This article offers a concise self-paced approach to help the individual nurse and/or smaller health care facility deliver optimal EBP nursing care to those within their range

Funding sources: None.
Conflict of interest: None.
Infection Prevention/Quality, Methodist Hospital for Surgery, 17101 North Dallas Parkway, Addison, TX 75001, USA
E-mail address: pgrant@methodistsurg.com

Perioperative Nursing Clinics 7 (2012) 401–409
http://dx.doi.org/10.1016/j.cpen.2012.08.006
1556-7931/12/$ – see front matter © 2012 Elsevier Inc. All rights reserved.

of practice. With the vision of making EBP an accessible goal for the nurse in any practice setting, Internet-based references are included when possible. Not every nurse or facility needs to possess textbook nursing research capabilities, but the skills to determine the strength behind published EBP research, and what potential barriers are involved with successful implementation of continuous improvement to advance patient safety, are essential.

The question that should come to mind when considering nursing EBP is: "So what?" This same question is asked repeatedly before, throughout, and at the conclusion of any thesis investigation and study. As far back as the year 2000, the term EBP was considered a "buzz phrase" of the last decade,[2] indicating that EBP was becoming mainstream in nursing as far back as the early 1990s when one of nursing's major success stories—moving from heparin to saline flush for intravenous access— took hold.[3] Despite the stable pursuit of EBP, one theme that becomes evident during a literature search involves facilitating the bedside nurse's ability to both understand and implement this critical health care research–oriented skill to provide optimal, productive, and/or cost-effective patient care.[2,4–6]

Health care facilities working toward and/or are successful Magnet Designation[7] sites must not only be conversant in EBP, but must also document consistent application, with progression of successful outcomes, based on their nursing-driven interventions. This valuable Magnet journey comes with a price tag upward of $23,000[8] based on 6 types of fees and appraiser(s) expenses. If a facility does not have the financial or university-affiliated resources to pursue the elite Magnet Designation, what other focused drivers are available to help achieve a solid EBP nursing program to provide optimal nursing care and patient safety for their patient population? The EBP Triangular Approach Toward Improvement Starter Kit, presented within this article (**Fig. 1**), is one option to foster published nursing research integration into clinical practice at the bedside, regardless of facility size or resources.

NURSING EBP IMPLEMENTATION STARTER KIT: A 3-PRONGED TRIANGULAR APPROACH
Side One: What Research to Quote when Implementing EBP Change

Side one of The EBP Triangular Approach Toward Improvement (The EBP Triangular Approach) is knowing what on-line reference(s) is/are robust enough to support EBP change at the bedside. Lack of access to a medical library should no longer be a major impediment to engaging in EBP nursing, because much of what is needed for the uncomplicated improvement process is available via the Internet.[4] Although not 100% inclusive, **Table 1** provides well-referenced Web sites to aid evidence-based nursing practice realization. These sources provide research to improve bedside practice when implementing an EBP approach to secure safe patient outcomes, while not disallowing astute resource management decisions that are monetary-based or based on human resources.

Some of the process improvement, EBP information, and university-affiliated Web sites in **Table 1** require a password; however, the publically accessible information includes self-paced tutorials, links to more EBP Web sites, and succinct approaches to EBP implementation. Many of the Internet-based resources included in **Table 1** are free of charge; however, it is best to include article download fees as part a generic nursing budget. Sometimes only the abstract of a peer-reviewed article is free, and the abstract itself might be insufficient to determine if the findings are applicable to your patient population and circumstances.

Cost estimation for untoward outcomes can be a frustration for the hands-on nurse. Trying to implement EBP at the bedside, without easy access to internal financial cost

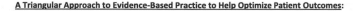

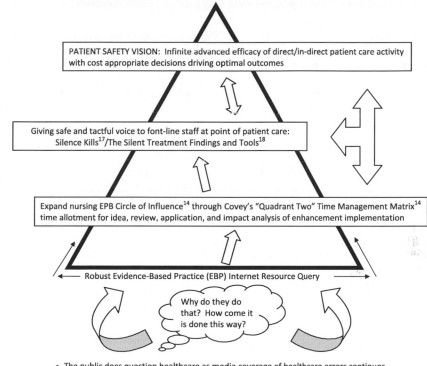

A Triangular Approach to Evidence-Based Practice to Help Optimize Patient Outcomes:

Nursing **Practice** Based on Published Peer-Reviewed Standards and/or Guidelines

- The public does question healthcare as media coverage of healthcare errors continues
- Nurses should advocate by questioning the nursing 'status quo' of patient care dynamics

Fig. 1. A triangular approach to evidence-based practice to help optimize patient outcomes: nursing practice based on published peer-reviewed standards and/or guidelines. The public does question health care as media coverage of health care errors continues. Nurses should advocate by questioning the nursing status quo of patient care dynamics.

resources that provide institution-specific cost determinations on patient falls, medication errors, or health care–associated infections (HAIs)[9] can impede resource justification for improvement. Disappointment can also mount when trying to "make current" cost estimations quoted in peer-reviewed articles. Examples of easy online tools to help customize the references found during the literature review to meet your facility activity includes: (1) The Inflation Calculator,[10] providing several options to bring cost quotes into current economic realities; and (2) the APIC (Association for Professionals in Infection Control and Epidemiology, Inc) health care–associated infection cost calculator,[11] which includes a downloadable file that can help estimate the cost of projected or known infections.

Practice makes perfect where familiarity with reading and critiquing research is concerned; however, there are some general rules for the novice to avoid, such as knowing what not to quote as a reference.[12,13] With rare exception, avoid using a reference that is not from a peer-reviewed journal, as these publications have been scrutinized by like-peers for scientific rigor and are coordinated by an experienced Editorial Review Board. Although newsletters, vanity publications, and magazines can provide good supplemental information, when providing documentation for change a peer-reviewed source is the gold standard.

Table 1 Internet evidence-based practice (EBP) Web sites: references for science-driven change and ideas to help implement change at the bedside to improve patient outcomes[a]	
Intellectual Source and/or EBP Clearinghouse	**Web Site Uniform Resources Locator (URL)**
http://www.guideline.gov/index.aspx EBP guidelines/literature Search	*Agency for Healthcare Research and Quality (AHRQ) National Guideline Clearinghouse*: public resource for evidence-based clinical practice guidelines
http://www.cdc.gov/hicpac/index.html EBP guidelines/literature Search	A Centers for Disease Control and Prevention Resource: *Health care Infection Control Practices Advisory Committee* (HICPAC): public resource for infection prevention and control strategies of health care–associated infections in United States health care facilities
http://www.ahrq.gov/clinic/epcindex.htm EBP guidelines/literature Search	AHRQ *Evidence-Based Practice Centers (EPCs)* topics via partnerships of professional societies, health plans, insurers, employers, and patient groups (A–Z listing)
http://www.thecochranelibrary.com/view/0/ index.html EBP guidelines/literature search reviews	*The Cochrane Collaboration* is an internatIonally recognized summary review of publications of EBP: http://www.cochrane-handbook.org/ provides free information
http://info.med.yale.edu/library/nursing/ education/ebresources.html University-based nursing EBP information	Yale University: Nursing EBP Resources
http://guides.library.vcu.edu/content.php? pid=121624&sid=1046039 University-based nursing EBP information	Virginia Commonwealth University: Nursing EBP Resources
http://ebp.lib.uic.edu/nursing/?q=node/12 University-based nursing EPB information	University of Illinois at Chicago: Nursing EBP Resources
http://www.cochranejournalclub.com/ The Cochrane Journal Club	Administered and maintained by The Cochrane Collaboration
http://www.brighthub.com/office/project- management/articles/97846.aspx#. The BRIGHT HUB: The Hub for Bright Minds	Free template for Plan, Do, Check, Act (PDCA) performance improvement model

[a] Examples are not inclusive and designed as a starting point.

Side Two: Making Time to Research EBP, Implement Findings, and Analyze Progress

Like most worthwhile endeavors, a large time allotment is required, and the continuous assessment of nursing EBP for the improvement of patient safety is no exception. Side two of The EBP Triangular Approach involves stating the obvious of "make time," yet not as a glib statement making light of the realities of concurrent demands within health care. Not surprisingly, the concept of expanding a nurse's "Circle of Influence" as coached by Stephen R. Covey[14] is much of what EBP in nursing is about.

Nurses, like other people, are concerned about many things (Circle of Concern[14]) yet must keep these multiple stimuli in perspective and determine which concerns they can affect through their Circle of Influence.[14] Once a nurse and/or multidisciplinary team makes the determination to influence change, thus expanding their Circle of Influence, and improve patient safety through EBP references, the challenge of time management still reigns supreme when compared with the pressing demands of real-time patient care. Like most health care professionals, nurses are faced with the prioritization demands of direct patient care when making the time for process improvement.

Covey developed "The Time Management Matrix,"[14] which can be applied to the importance of managing time for EBP implementation in nursing, no matter how limited the perceived resources of the individual or team affecting the change of improved patient care. The urgency of real-time patient needs can create a false environmental dilemma of needlessly living in what Covey deems "Quadrant One" where things important and urgent require immediate action. In nursing there exist real Quadrant One situations such as Code Blue, patient fall, wrong-site surgery, medication error, or not addressing a low potassium level before surgery; however, without managing time for analysis of these true Quadrant One episodes, working outside of Quadrant One can become a lofty goal. Without examination of the circumstances surrounding these important and urgent occurrences, and implementation and feedback checks of findings for improvement, these situations may not decline unless processes are examined for prevention of occurrence and/or improvement of systemic procedures.

Securing time for improvement through the review and application of the EBP nursing required within your health care facility entails managing human resource "time" within Quadrant Two (important and nonurgent) of Covey's Time Management Matrix.[14] The quandary is making this happen, as there is no magic bullet or panacea. Stating the necessity for Quadrant Two planning is a fact that must be secured via support of health care administration for time allotment away from direct patient care, by those that provide that same direct patient care.

One approach is to make a brief a presentation that states: (1) here are the free resources (see **Table 1**) that we have accessed; (2) to apply to this challenge; and (3) what is required for success of patient safety improvement is support for front-line professionals to have time away from the bedside to engage in planning to make this happen.[15,16] This approach may feel uncomfortable as it requires a commitment to processes that are novel, and once approved for implementation the time-management allotments must be honored for long-reaching success to happen.

Side Three: Create a Safe Place for the Adoption of a Nursing EBP Milieu

After 30 years in health care witnessing and participating in multiple improvement projects, it seems it is one thing to know what to do (willingness) and a vastly different thing to be repetitively successful (ability). It is doubtful that this is deliberate; health care professionals do not go to work thinking "I am going to deliberately harm a patient today." Indeed, consistent implementation struggles are not unique to health care, yet the ingrained hierarchal communication patterns seem to be impeding progress,[17] leading to the purpose of side three of the triangle. Side three of The EBP Triangular Approach involves creating awareness first, and then working toward a culture of safety, to promote the willingness and ability of bedside staff to "do the right thing" on a consistent basis as one team functioning in unison.

The complexities involved with accurate and candid communication have been given a recent voice in health care. Conducted by VitalSmarts and the American Association of Critical Care Nurses (AACN), the publication SILENCE KILLS[17] is the first of 2 studies examining communication patterns and the impact on patient care. Released in 2005, this study of 1700 health care professionals with varying levels of responsibility and expertise illustrates what can happen when there is silence about noncompliance with established standards of care. The subjective opinion of these health care workers regarding their objective conclusions of "seeing and not telling or interfering at various levels" with potentially harmful behaviors of fellow health care providers gives one pause.

The publication examines 7 perceived areas of specific health care cultural realities that are involved with medical errors, patient safety, quality of care, employee satisfaction, staff commitment, and turnover. Even though more than half of the respondents eventually took responsibility by reporting situations up the chain of command, the self-reported method of communication approximately 90% of the time was of not confronting the individual head-on, at the actual time of the observed potentially harmful action. Stated another way, 10% of participants felt empowered to halt the purportedly harmful activities of a fellow coworker immediately, with the direct result of feeling they improved patient outcome. So how does a person or organization move this 10% closer to 100%?

Prevalence of the 7 most crucial concerns studied—Broken Rules, Mistakes, Lack of Support, Incompetence, Poor Teamwork, Disrespect, and Micromanagement—can be daunting, if not overwhelming, for cultural reversal to promote feelings of trust and support to "do the right thing" without repercussions from the political arena(s) in health care. SILENCE KILLS does include a succinct action plan for moving forward, including recruitment of the 10% "skilled minority"[17] to serve as living examples of successful advocacy of patient safety.

In 2010, the follow-up study included the collaboration of The Association of periOperative Registered Nurses (AORN), and studied 2383 nurses of a convenience sample to examine the "undiscussables" that can impede the successful implementation of check-lists[18] that are driven by EBP. Echoing the 2005 publication findings,[17] the 3 main areas of concern examined in the report, *The Silent Treatment*,[18] include dangerous shortcuts, incompetence, and disrespect. One fascinating and insightful aspect of the 2010 document are direct quotes from the participants describing observations and the impact of their actions.

As with the 2005 publication, the 2010 follow-up study also includes references for the development of action plans to help move an organization toward a culture of safety by using a multifaceted approach toward being able to discuss the "undiscussables" in general. This must be an ever-present goal, especially when considering that 4 of 5 participants stated concerns around the "undiscussables."[18] Another study admittance that can help a facility feel a sense of urgency in creating a culture of safety is that 1 in 4 respondents admitted to having seen shortcuts or incompetence result in patient harm.[18]

Personal experience has taught the author to state the obvious when working with those in doubt of their own empowerment contributions to promoting a culture of safety. Hand hygiene is a common and required activity in infection-prevention guidelines,[19,20] yet reliable compliance remains a safety issue in health care facilities. The next time you observe an employee ignore it when a fellow health care professional does not clean their hands, ask them why. When they share "fearful of the person going to administration to complain" or "I can't make a difference as just one person," try the following interactive exercise.

Anecdotally speaking, the exchange below has been successful in the author's 20 years of functioning as an infection preventionist. After you get the above response to the question "why didn't you say something," respond: "What is the worst that can happen?" Think about how this will play out if a complaint is filed:

1. You tactfully remind the person to clean his or her hands in a manner that does not alarm the patient or embarrass your coworker; so,

2. As long as you are tactful and professional your behavior shouldn't be questioned or result in a complaint to administration; therefore,
3. If they go to administration and complain "Nurse Grant told me to wash my hands before inserting a central line (or changing a dressing, or inserting a urinary catheter, or leaving an isolation room)"... can you imagine how that conversation might progress?
4. The administrator, at some point, must state the obvious: "Are you bringing me a complaint that Nurse Grant told you to clean your hands before patient care? What am I supposed to do, tell him or her not to worry about spreading infection? That it is acceptable to give the patient extra pain and suffering with an infection?"

Affirming this simple role-playing dialogue often made the light bulb go on when the person mentally followed through on their imagined and feared administrative complaint voiced by a person thought to be more powerful. "One person at a time," over many years, has helped empower others toward corrective behavioral action—not a scientific correlation by any means, yet a technique that has helped others secure their role in making their facility safer.

THE EBP NURSING CHALLENGE OF PERPETUAL MOTION

The crunch of weighted recommendations, based on the strength of the science within nursing practice, was in full swing at the close of the last century. Even the admired AORN Perioperative Standards and Recommended Practices, which traditionally enjoyed a challenge-free implementation environment, is embracing the EBP approach to provide their membership with the strength of robust scientific-backed rationale for their guideline implementation.[21] Application of EBP in nursing must start somewhere, and sometimes the literature search does not provide enough evidence, and a preliminary publication must be produced[22] to encourage validation or application studies. Another purpose of EBP nursing is to ground all practices in science whenever possible, leading the way to eliminate the practice of routine patient care simply because it was always done that way.[23]

No matter which angle of emphasis you choose for your EBP nursing journey, know that it must be done in a format that can track progress, identify unanticipated setbacks, provide an opportunity to reassess, and examine efficacy of implementations. Although most facilities have at least one quality improvement professional to use as their guiding resource, this EBP Triangular Approach Starter Kit would be incomplete without sharing one process-improvement model. The PDCA Model (Plan, Do, Check, Act) is established, and when used properly can provide proactive outcomes when used concurrently throughout the change process; moreover, an online resource is offered for consideration.[24]

Whether in a large or small health care facility, nurses must keep challenging themselves to provide the best scientific-based practice to those who entrust their lives to the health care system: our patients and their loved ones. The starter kit presented with this article (see **Fig. 1**) is designed to help smaller facilities and critical access hospitals[25] begin or expand a program to keep EBP current within their bedside nursing practice. The angles of The Evidence-Based Practice Triangular Approach Toward Improvement involve:

- Seeking out and referencing robust referenced literature (see **Table 1**) to implement safer patient care, while
- Expanding the Circle of Influence[14] while securing time in Quadrant Two of Covey's Time Management Matrix[14]

- And working toward a culture of safety through the lessons learned and shared by others[17,18]

This suggested triangular approach to implementing EBP is designed as "one-stop shopping" to help smaller facilities get an EBP program off the ground, yet is shared with the hope that content presented might provide a stimulus for EBP enhancement efforts of larger facilities. Without all the sides of a triangle it cannot stand, and should provide a visualization of the importance of considering not just the references involved with EBP, but the time allotment to foster change, while assessing and establishing a culture of safety.

REFERENCES

1. PubMed (US National Library of Medicine. National Institutes of Health). Available at: http://www.ncbi.nlm.nih.gov/sites/entrez. Accessed May 1, 2012.
2. Beyea SC. Why should perioperative RNs care about evidence-based practice? AORN J 2000;72:109–11.
3. Good CJ, Titler M, Rakel B, et al. A meta-analysis of effects of heparin flush and saline flush: quality and cost implications. Nurs Res 1991;40(6):314–30.
4. Hoss B, Hanson D. Evaluating the evidence: web sites. AORN J 2008;87:124–41.
5. Luby M, Riley JK, Towne G. Nursing research journal clubs: bridging the gap between practice and research. Medsurg Nurs 2006;15:100–2.
6. Windle PE. Understanding evidence-based practice. J Perianesth Nurs 2003;18: 360–2.
7. American Nurses Credentialing Center Magnet Recognition Program®. Available at: http://nursecredentialing.org/Magnet.aspx. Accessed May 1, 2012.
8. American Nurses Credentialing Center Magnet Recognition Program® Schedule of Fees. Available at: http://nursecredentialing.org/MagnetScheduleFees.aspx. Accessed May 1, 2012.
9. Stone PW, Hedblom EC, Murphy DM. The economic impact of infection control: making the business case for increased infection control resources. Am J Infect Control 2005;33:542–7.
10. InflationData.com. Your place in cyber space for inflation data. Available at: http://inflationdata.com/Inflation/Inflation_Calculators/Inflation_Rate_Calculator.asp. Accessed May 6, 2012.
11. Association for Professionals in Infection Control and Epidemiology, Inc. Healthcare-associated infection cost calculators. Available at: http://www.apic.org/Resources/Cost-calculators. Accessed May 6, 2012.
12. Lacovara JE. When searching for evidence, stop using Wikipedia. Medsurg Nurs 2008;17:153.
13. Hanson D, Hoss BL, Wesorick B. Evaluating the evidence: guidelines. AORN J 2008;88:184–96.
14. Covey SR. The 7 habits of highly effective people: powerful lessons in personal change. New York: Free Press; 1989. p. 67–94, 146–82.
15. Segel K. Thinking big: the world's great organizations may hold the key to a more compelling business case for HAI elimination. Prevention strategist. Spring 2010. Available at: http://valuecapturellc.com/ps1001.pdf. Accessed May 6, 2012.
16. Segel K. Saving lives saving money: helping hospital leaders seize the opportunity. Prevention strategist. Summer 2010. Available at: http://valuecapturellc.com/ps1002.pdf. Accessed May 7, 2012.

17. Maxfield D, Grenny J, McMillan R, et al. SILENCE KILLS: the seven crucial con-versations® for healthcare. 2005. Available at: http://www.silenttreatmentstudy.com/silencekills/SilenceKills.pdf. Accessed May 6, 2012.

18. Maxfield D, Grenny J, Lavandero R, et al. The silent treatment: why safety tools and checklists aren't enough to save lives. 2010. Available at: http://www.silenttreatmentstudy.com/silent/The%20Silent%20Treatment.pdf. Accessed May 7, 2012.

19. Boyce JM, Pittet D. Morbidity and Mortality Weekly Report Guideline for hand hygiene in health-care settings: recommendations of the healthcare infection control practices advisory committee and the HICPAC/SHEA/APIC/IDSA hand hygiene task force. 2002. Available at: http://www.cdc.gov/mmwr/PDF/rr/rr5116.pdf. Accessed May 7, 2012.

20. World Health Organization. WHO guidelines in hand hygiene in healthcare. 2009. Available at: http://whqlibdoc.who.int/publications/2009/9789241597906_eng.pdf. Accessed May 7, 2012.

21. Steelman VM, Pape T, King CA, et al. Selection of a method to rate the strength of scientific evidence for AORN recommendations. AORN J 2011;93:433–44.

22. Grant PS, Charns LG, Rawot BW, et al. Consideration to culture health care workers related to increased methicillin-resistant *Staphylococcus aureus* activity in a neonatal intensive care unit. Am J Infect Control 2008;36:638–43.

23. Mellinger E, McCanless L. Evidence-based nursing practice in the perioperative setting: a magnet journey to eliminate sacred cows. AORN J 2010;92:572–8.

24. Levine R. Attacking issues with the PDCA process: free template for down-load. 2011. Available at: http://www.brighthub.com/office/project-management/articles/97846.aspx#. Accessed May 7, 2012.

25. Rural Assistance Center: health and human services information for rural America. Available at: http://www.raconline.org/topics/hospitals/cahfaq.php http://www.raconline.org/topics/hospitals/cah.php. Accessed May 7, 2012.

Advocating for Perioperative Learning Through Learning Practice Communities

Andrea E. Berndt, PhD[a],*, Evelyn Swenson-Britt, PhD, RN[b],
Rosemary K. Rushmer, PhD[c]

KEYWORDS

- Perioperative units • Learning practice communities • Research efficacy
- Professional practice environment

KEY POINTS

- This article considers barriers to nurses' collective learning in perioperative units and suggests the development of learning practice communities as a potential solution.
- Several characteristics of learning practice communities are identified and strategies to encourage their development in perioperative units are proposed.

PERIOPERATIVE UNITS AS LEARNING PRACTICE COMMUNITIES

Perioperative nursing is one of the longest-established specialties in nursing practice.[1] During the 1960s, perioperative nurses increased their focus on patient safety and excellence in the delivery of patient care.[2] Nurses who choose perioperative nursing for their specialty area intertwine the roles of clinician, technician, trouble shooter, and educator in their nursing practice. As one of their responsibilities is to maintain a safe environment, perioperative nurses act as the primary patient advocate during a time in which patients cannot speak for themselves.[3] Among the reasons why perioperative nurses often remain in the specialty area throughout their careers is the satisfaction they gain from one-on-one nurse-patient relationships, and from knowing they performed their tasks in the way they believe tasks should be done.[4]

Disclosure Statement: None of the authors have financial relationships to commercial companies that have direct financial relationships to the subject matter in this article.
Note: There are no drug or equipment trademarks appearing in this article.
[a] School of Nursing, Family and Community Health Systems Department, The University of Texas Health Science Center at San Antonio, 7703 Floyd Curl Drive MC 7950, San Antonio, TX 78229, USA; [b] Center for Excellence in Patient Care, University Health System, 4502 Medical Drive, San Antonio, TX 78229, USA; [c] School of Health and Social Care, Teesside University, School of Health and Social Care, Vicarage Road, Darlington DL1 1JW, Middlesbrough, Yorkshire TS1 3BA, United Kingdom
* Corresponding author.
E-mail address: Berndt@uthscsa.edu

Perioperative Nursing Clinics 7 (2012) 411–424
http://dx.doi.org/10.1016/j.cpen.2012.08.008
1556-7931/12/$ – see front matter © 2012 Elsevier Inc. All rights reserved.
periopnursing.theclinics.com

The delivery of excellent patient care is dependent on a work environment that advocates for a learning environment. Among the organizations important to perioperative nurses, the Association of PeriOperative Registered Nurses set several goals to promote quality and increase the use of evidence-based standards in patient care.[5] These goals require nurses to implement these standards in a challenging, fast-paced practice setting with multiple team members. Moreover, it also necessitates continual reading and evaluation of the latest evidence-based research findings to implement best practices in perioperative settings.

Research on successful learning practices has long suggested that much can be gained by the following:

- Practice teams encouraged to reflect on their practice and learn together[6–8];
- Changes initiated by practitioners for themselves (rather than imposed)[9,10];
- Sustainable innovations focused on quality improvements[11–13];
- A greater appreciation of the role of fellow practitioners and a holistic appreciation of the system of care delivery[14–16];
- Development of ongoing resilience in spite of the constant "churn" involved in the delivery of health care services.[17,18]

Beyond these benefits, there is a more pragmatic reason to encourage practitioner-led change. The pressure of constantly changing technologies, treatments, and patient demands means that the current delivery of services (even if excellent now) will ultimately become dated. The ability to be flexible, to support innovation and to promote continual learning is likely to be as important as any individual profession-based skill.[19,20] The challenge is how to prompt and support these characteristics at the front line of service delivery.

UNDERSTANDING THE PERIOPERATIVE WORK ENVIRONMENT
Is Yours an Impetus or Obstacle to Learning?

It makes sense that the provision of safe, effective, patient care within a complex work environment requires perioperative nurses to learn new skills and knowledge. Conversely, it is imperative that nurses also understand cultural and psychological factors that influence the persistence of unsafe nursing practices and that interfere with learning in interdisciplinary teams.[21] These factors have been shown to negatively affect the learning culture of an organization.[22] Because of the severity of consequences from errors in the operating room (OR), the need for improved safety is urgent and depends on creating a climate that supports teamwork and collective learning.[23]

The "vulnerable system syndrome" occurs when health care organizations use blame, denial, and/or pursuit of financial gains to promote changes in behavior, rather than by focusing on patient safety or excellence.[24] Characteristics of this syndrome include targeting individual health care professionals for poor patient outcomes, dismissing the presence of organizational factors related to systematic errors, and an overreliance on numerical indices tied to financial performance. Although a hyperfocus on the financial performance of perioperative units is not wise, it is also not surprising. One study indicated that the operating room in many hospitals generates up to 70% of hospital revenues, but also accounts for 20% to 40% of hospital costs.[25]

Interestingly, when surgeons, anesthesiologists, and perioperative nurses were asked to identify causes of hypothetical error scenarios within the operating room, their responses most often identified individual rather than systemic failures.[26] For example, they identified the presence of a retained sponge postsurgery, administration of Ancef to an allergic patient, and a burned bile duct as causes of error; however, they rarely identified demands to maintain an OR schedule, requirements for multi-tasking, or other system issues as underlying causes of error. Consistent with the vulnerable system syndrome, they indicated the appropriate response to these hypothetical scenarios was individual remediation. This reaction is problematic because it encourages a culture of blame, rather than promoting a culture of observation, inquiry, and discussion.[26]

Another factor that interferes with improvement of safe patient care delivery was noted in nurses' willingness to report incidents that occurred within the OR. Given the errors identified for the scenarios, OR nurses indicated they would report 61% and would use an incident report for 45%.[27] Nurses indicated they would most likely informally report the incident and share the information in their break room. The choice to report these incidents informally rather than formally, further isolates potential sources of error by limiting communication and opportunities for learning.

Tucker and Edmondson[28] refer to this reaction as first-order problem solving, in which the nurse responds to problems with a "work around" or "quick fix" but avoids addressing the fundamental cause. Second-order problem solving involves sharing of errors and working as a team to find root causes and effect solutions to prevent their reoccurrence. In a work environment that encourages second-order problem solving, leadership provides nurses with a clear understanding of the individual's importance within the team and the authority to ensure errors are seen as an opportunity to improve their practice.

An innovative approach to addressing these barriers to learning in clinical nursing units is to create learning practice communities or communities of practice.[29–32] The characteristics of learning practice communities include encouraging members to identify existing or potential problems, to apply and evaluate solutions, and to reflect on those results individually and collectively. The development of learning practice communities has been successful in promoting work environments in which engaged, confident employees routinely share information and develop new knowledge.[32]

In such a work environment, nurses could focus on challenges to their clinical practice and act on shared knowledge and expertise to enhance quality patient care. Nurses and other team members could implement and evaluate best practices by keeping abreast of the latest published research. Unfortunately, to date, research on and application of research on learning practice communities in perioperative settings has been extremely limited.[26]

A BRIEF HISTORY OF LEARNING PRACTICE COMMUNITIES IN HEALTH CARE SETTINGS
The Journey Begins in the United Kingdom

In the early 2000s, discussions began between professionals from the NHS Education for Scotland[33] and academics at St Andrews University in Scotland (written communication, Rosemary Rushmer, PhD, March 2012). Early work focused on what it would take to prompt the development of general practices (ie, primary care teams based in the community, composed of general practitioners, nurses, allied health professionals, and administrative staff) to foster units that were capable of collectively learning and steering their ongoing practice development. A literature review was undertaken and a series of position papers were produced.[29–31] These position papers reviewed theories of learning organizations, organizational learning, and communities of practice, as well as empiric findings about how these concepts had been applied and tested in health care settings. They detailed the characteristics of learning practices, and the actions necessary to develop them, the core contextual factors necessary to support them, and what learning practices might be able to achieve. They defined a learning practice as

> A G(eneral) P(ractice) (or similar) unit where individual, collective and organizational learning and development is systematically pursued according to Learning Organization principles, to enhance service provision in a way that is increasingly satisfying to its patients, staff and other stakeholders.[29]

This work was published as a trilogy of articles.[29–31] A key finding from these articles was that collective learning works best when it is generated by front-line staff, because they most often pursue learning that is directly relevant for their practice and the care of patients. A second insight was that the capacity to learn collectively is heavily influenced by contextual and cultural factors. Overall, strategies that placed "control" of proactive change with front-line staff resulted in changes that were more realistic, more focused on service needs, and sustained over longer periods of time.

Use of Learning Practice Communities in Nursing

Nurses must continuously adopt, change, learn, and ensure new methods of cutting-edge patient care delivery. Patient outcomes and research findings provide a daily stream of new knowledge about changes in health care. How do practicing nurses maintain skills and knowledge competencies? How do nurses practicing in complex clinical nursing units incorporate new knowledge into their practice? Moreover, if learning practice communities are developed within clinical nursing units, how would they function?

The ability to answer these questions is constrained by limited knowledge and research in this area. A recent systematic review of health and business literature reinforced the paucity of research on communities of practice in health care settings.[26] To conduct their review, the authors hand-searched key journals (eg, the *Journal of Continuing Education in Health Care* and *Harvard Business Review*), examined reference lists from articles and books published from 1991 to 2005, and searched electronic databases. They examined how communities of practice as described by Lave and Wenger[34] were defined in business and health care settings. Only 26 articles were identified in health care settings. Of these, 13 were primary studies. Unfortunately, none of these studies met criteria for inclusion because they lacked quantitative analyses.

A review of the literature on learning practices located a single study that focused on nurses in a postanesthesia care setting.[26] This qualitative study took place over a span of 1.5 years and sampled 32 nurses. The aims of the study were (1) to elicit information from nurses about how they learn and solve problems; and (2) to gather nurses' descriptions about the influence from nursing knowledge to patient outcomes. Beyond links between nursing knowledge and patient outcomes, nursing knowledge also linked to work-based learning and collaborative competence. Collaborative competence was defined as nurses' ability to work and learn collectively. These findings support the importance of collaborative learning to manage rapid changes and to use information to achieve positive patient outcomes.

The Learning Practice Inventory

Based on recurrent themes and concept statements extracted from the position papers on learning practices, the Learning Practice Inventory (LPI) was developed to assess characteristics of learning practices in health care settings.[29–31,35] The original LPI is composed of 62 randomly placed items, scored on a bipolar scale, using a response scale that ranges from 1 to 10 (data on the psychometric qualities of the original LPI can be obtained from NHS Education for Scotland). On bipolar scales, participants are asked to identify the closest match to their attitudes on a scale between 2 divergent adjectives or statements (eg, Happy-Sad, or Exhausted-Energetic). Organization of related concept statements across the LPI can be used to categorize each item into 1 of 3 primary scales: Engagement, Support, and Learning (see **Table 1** for descriptions).

The LPI collects data on how practitioners perceive their team functions (eg, behaviors, attitudes, culture, structures, and processes). The LPI was designed to identify the presence of learning techniques and contextual factors that might facilitate or impede collective learning. These data can then serve as a developmental tool to (1) to determine how closely these perceptions align with a learning practice; and (2) to consider how easily the team might learn or change collectively.[29–31]

Data from the LPI are not designed to measure or evaluate the effectiveness of a given change initiative. Instead, the LPI data assesses the underlying capacity of a team to learn and change practice. Ideally, data from the LPI provide feedback for teams to evaluate their current level of reflective practice and to build capacity for change while maintaining "business as usual."[29–31]

Evaluating Nurses' Perceptions about Learning Practice Communities in the United States

In a recent dissertation, Swenson-Britt[36] assessed practicing nurses' perceptions about the degree to which characteristics of learning practice communities were present in their clinical nursing units, using a cross-sectional survey design. Although many research questions were investigated in this dissertation, the current article limits discussion to those that are directly relevant to learning practice communities. The questions of interest include the following: (1) To what extent do nurses perceive that characteristics of learning communities are present in their clinical units? (2) Are these perceptions influenced by characteristics of the nurses, such as their education or number of years in a nursing position? (3) Are these perceptions influenced by ratings about individual nursing units as professional practice environments? (4) Are positive perceptions of a nursing unit as a learning practice community related to higher research self-efficacy, higher collective research-efficacy, and increased reports of research behavior?

Table 1		
Learning Practice Inventory (LPI) domains and definitions		
LPI Domain	**No. Items[a]**	**Definition**
Engagement	15 (14)	The extent to which nurses exhibit ownership, involvement, supportive attitudes and beliefs that collective learning is safe and expected in the organization.
Learning	25 (21)	The extent to which nurses develop and persist in collective learning routines to share and search for knowledge, clinical expertise, and problem solving, resulting in process improvements and positive outcomes.
Support	22 (20)	The extent to which organizational resources, education and training, information, and information systems support nurses' behaviors to learn collectively.
Total	62 (55)	

[a] Total number of items on the original LPI (total number of items on the modified LPI).

Participants were 231 practicing nurses from 10 nursing units (medical-surgical, intensive care, intermediate care, rehabilitation, diagnostic testing) within an academic medical center (AMC). Participants were asked to complete a modified-LPI, the Nurse Research Self-Efficacy Scale (NURSES),[37] a 6-item measure to assess the frequency in which they engaged in research behaviors and to provide demographics (ie, highest level of education, number of years in nursing, and their nursing unit). NURSES is a 38-item instrument that measures participants' degree of research self-efficacy and their perceptions about their unit's collective research efficacy. Items that measure research self-efficacy are further categorized into 4 subscales that can iden-tify strengths of limitations in specific research areas (see **Table 2** for NURSES subscales and range of scores).

To assess perceptions about clinical nursing units as professional practice environ-ments, the average scores from the last 2 years' registered nurse (RN) satisfaction survey, Practice Environment Scale-Nursing Work Index (PES-NWI),[38,39] were exam-ined for all nursing units within the AMC. The PES-NWI yields 5 subscale scores and a total, using a 4-point scale in which 1 = extreme dissatisfaction and 4 = extreme satisfaction. The 5 subscales examine satisfaction with (1) participation in organization governance, (2) foundations of quality care, (3) nursing leadership, (4) staffing, and (5) collegial nurse-physician relationships.

Benchmark data are given along with unit scores for PES-NWI subscale and total scores to allow for comparisons to similar unit types (ie, critical care, obstetrics, medical-surgical) and similar organizational structures. Based on unit comparisons to their appropriate comparisons, unit scores can be categorized as representing practice environments that are above average, average, or below average. The 10 nursing units that participated in this study were chosen to be representative across

Table 2
Nurses Research Self-Efficacy Scale subscales, descriptions, number of items, and range of possible scores

Subscale	Description	# Items	Range of Possible Scores
Obtain Resources[a]	Ability to obtain and critically evaluate resources	6	6–30
Qualitative Research[a]	Ability to read and critically evaluate qualitative research literature	7	7–35
Quantitative Research[a]	Ability to read and critically evaluate quantitative research literature	6	6–30
Understand/Apply Theory[a]	Ability to understand and apply theory to different research contexts	9	9–45
Collective Research-Efficacy[b]	Perceptions about the degree to which nurses in a unit engage in activities that facilitate research engagement	10	10–50
Total		38	

[a] These subscales measure research self-efficacy.
[b] This subscale measures collective research-efficacy.

PES-NWI categorizations, the number of assigned RNs, and patient populations cared for in different units.

Permission to modify and use the LPI for this study was obtained from the primary author of the instrument. Five nurses participated in conducting an initial assessment and review of the original instrument to determine its usability and clarity for nurses in the United States. The nurses read through the LPI and were asked to express concerns they had with an item such as, but not limited to, confusion, length, and/or terminology. Across the LPI, 37 (60%) items were identified as confusing based on their context, use, or familiarity. This review led to removal of 7 items that were deemed inappropriate for nurses practicing in the United States.

Additionally, based on the nurses' feedback, the LPI was further modified in 3 ways. First, the introduction to the LPI was modified to explain its design, to provide an example for nurses' responses, and to focus it toward clinical nursing units. Second, items on the LPI were presented within the 3 primary scales to create an organized structure and to decrease the likelihood of respondent burden and stress associated with completing lengthy instruments. Finally, the response scale was modified from 1 to 10 to 1 to 9 to create mathematically identical distances between each pair of statements. See **Table 3** for a breakdown of the modified-LPI scales, subscales, and range of possible scores. Following all modifications, the revised 55-item LPI was resubmitted to the primary author (Dr. Rushmer) to ensure the remaining concept statements were consistent with the LPI's theoretical framework.

Several interesting findings were noted in the results.[36] **Table 4** presents mean scores, SDs, and minimum and maximum values for nurses' responses to subscales on the LPI and NURSES. A review of these values indicates that overall, mean scores were relatively high (from the 72nd to the 78th percentile) across the LPI with the exception of 2 subscales. Specifically, on the primary scale of Support, 2 subscales, *Structure* and *Behaviors*, had substantially lower scores (from the 60th to the 64th percentile).

In general, the mean scores on the NURSES subscales were substantially lower than those on the LPI. Specifically, among the 4 Research Self-Efficacy subscales, *Qualitative Research* had the lowest scores (slightly lower than the 50th percentile) whereas *Obtain Resources* had the highest scores (the 68th percentile). Mean scores for the Collective Research Efficacy subscale were also lower (slightly lower than the 60th percentile).

Overall, nurses reported relatively low engagement in research behaviors (**Table 5**). More than 50% reported they had not attended or presented at any local or national

Table 3
Learning Practice Inventory (LPI) domains and subdomains and range of possible scores

LPI Domain	LPI Subdomain	# Items	Range of Possible Scores
Engagement	Attitudes/Beliefs	8	8–72
	Ownership	6	6–45
Learning	Benefits	7	7–63
	Evidence	7	7–63
	Momentum	7	7–63
Support	Behaviors	6	6–45
	Structures	7	7–63
	Systems	7	7–63
Total		55	

Note: The modified-LPI was used to reflect the number of items in each LPI subdomain.

Table 4
Descriptive statistics for subscales of the Learning Practice Inventory (LPI) and Nurses
Research Self-Efficacy Scale (NURSES) (n = 231)

	Mean (SD)	Minimum	Maximum
LPI: *Engagement*			
Attitude/Beliefs	56.28 (11.76)	11	72
Ownership/Involvement	34.20 (7.69)	8	45
LPI: *Learning*			
Benefits	47.94 (9.97)	10	63
Evidence of Routines	45.64 (11.02)	11	63
Momentum	45.81 (11.08)	11	63
LPI: *Support*			
Behaviors	37.76 (10.45)	10	54
Structures	40.38 (12.55)	7	63
Systems/Practices	47.05 (10.27)	11	63
NURSES: *Research Self-Efficacy*			
Obtain Resources	20.32 (6.53)	6	30
Qualitative Research	17.03 (7.66)	7	35
Quantitative Research	16.84 (6.66)	6	30
Understand/Apply Theory	28.19 (9.29)	9	45
NURSES: *Collective Research Efficacy*	29.11 (10.54)	10	50

conferences in the past year. Further, about 50% reported they had not served in any research role in the past year. In contrast, slightly more than 40% indicated they spent an average of 1 to 2 hours each week reading research information. Also, almost 50% reported they shared research findings with peers once or twice in the past month.

Interestingly, the distribution of nurses who reported participating in 1 or 2 committees that used research findings in the past year was proportional to nurses who reported no participation in such (30% for both). Similar parity was also noted between the percentage of nurses who had not earned any Continuing Education (CE) credits focused on research, and those who earned 1 or 2 CE credits focused on research in the past 5 years (33% and 36%, respectively).

The most intriguing findings were noted in positive, significant relationships between all LPI subscales and all NURSES subscales (**Table 6**). Specifically, moderate, positive relationships were found between the LPI's *Engagement* and *Learning* subscales and *Research Self-Efficacy* subscales of the NURSES (*r* values ranging from 0.24 to 0.31). Positive relationships were also noted between the LPI's *Support* subscales and *Research Self-Efficacy* subscales of the NURSES, albeit with greater variability (*r* values ranging from 0.19 to 0.31). More importantly, all LPI subscales evidenced moderate or strong positive relationships to *Collective Research Efficacy* on the NURSES (*r* values from 0.38 to 0.53).

Finally, Swenson-Britt performed an exploratory analysis to investigate if units with nurses who reported the presence of more characteristics of learning practice communities differed from those in which few characteristics were reported.[36] One pattern was noted. That is, units that had scores at the 50th percentile or higher on the *Learning* subscales always had scores at the 50th percentile or higher on the *Support* subscales; however, no patterns were noted when units had scores at the 50th percentile or higher for either the *Engagement* or *Support* subscales. Further,

Table 5
Percentage and number of nurses engaging in research behaviors (n = 231)

Research Behavior	% (n)
Read research (weekly)	
Not at all	4.3 (10)
<1 h/wk	29.4 (68)
1–2 h/wk	42.4 (98)
3–5 h/wk	16.5 (38)
>5 h/wk	7.4 (17)
Serve in research roles (yearly)	
None	48.5 (112)
1–2 times/y	28.1 (65)
3–5 times/y	13.4 (31)
>5 times/y	10.0 (23)
Attend/present local conferences (yearly)	
None	53.7 (124)
1–2 times/y	38.5 (89)
3–5 times/y	4.8 (11)
>5 times/y	3.0 (7)
Obtain research CE credits (yearly)	
None	32.9 (76)
1 to 2 CE credits/y	35.5 (82)
3 to 5 CE credits/y	13.4 (31)
>5 CE credits/y	18.2 (42)
Share research with peers (monthly)	
None	39.8 (92)
Once or twice/mo	47.2 (109)
3–5 times/mo	9.5 (22)
>5 times/mo	3.5 (8)
Participate committees using research (yearly)	
None	32.9 (76)
1–2 times/y	32.5 (75)
3–5 times/y	16.9 (39)
>5 times/y	17.7 (41)
Attend/present national conferences (yearly)	
None	64.9 (150)
1–2 times/y	32.5 (75)
3–5 times/y	2.2 (5)
>5 times/y	0.4 (1)

when units had nurses who reported greater engagement in research behaviors, there was also a tendency for these units to have elevated *Learning* and *Support* scores. These findings may suggest the presence of support and learning characteristics is of greater importance to develop a learning practice community than is the initial presence of engagement characteristics.

This pattern was investigated at subsequent focus group sessions at the unit level. Nurses were asked to provide examples of positive learning experiences in their unit

Table 6
Relationships between Learning Practice Inventory (LPI) and Nurses Research Self-Efficacy Scale (NURSES) subscales (n = 231)

| | LPI | | | | | | | |
| | Engagement | | Learning | | | Support | | |
NURSES	Attitud	Ownrshp	Benft	Evdnc	Moment	Behav	Struct	Systm
Research Self-Efficacy								
Obtain Resources	.26	.34	.27	.25	.25	.21	.19	.25
Qualitative Research	.25	.28	.31	.30	.30	.31	.29	.27
Quantitative Research	.24	.27	.28	.26	.26	.28	.23	.28
Und/Apply Theory	.26	.29	.29	.26	.26	.29	.20	.25
Collective Resrch Eff	.41	.51	.52	.53	.47	.51	.38	.42

Note: All Pearson product-moment correlations are significant at 0.01 level (2-tailed).
Abbreviations: Attitud, Attitudes/Beliefs; Behav, Behaviors; Benft, Benefits; Collective Resrch Eff, Collective Research Efficacy; Evdnc, Evidence; Moment, Momentum; Ownrshp, Ownership; Struct, Structures; Systm, Systems; Und/Apply Theory, Understand/Apply Theory.

and then were given summary data about their unit as a learning practice community. Responses from sessions indicated that when nurses perceived their unit environment fostered questioning, encouraged professional development, provided accurate and readily accessible information, and facilitated respect and collaboration, they offered more examples of positive and frequent learning experiences. These comments mirrored many items from *Support* subscales (**Box 1**).

Collectively, the findings indicated that nurses who strongly identified characteristics of engagement, support, and learning in their units had greater research self-efficacy and collective research efficacy. Collective research efficacy was moderately or strongly correlated with all LPI subscales, suggesting collective research efficacy supports a culture for learning. These findings also suggest that engaging in research behaviors may serve as learning opportunities for nurses.

CREATING LEARNING PRACTICE COMMUNITIES IN PERIOPERATIVE UNITS

Within perioperative units, unit leaders and staff members can create a culture of learning. Learning practice communities can emerge if leaders and staff are willing to encourage systemic analysis of error and empower frontline staff to improve their practice.[29–31] Unit leaders and staff must have shared goals that foster the development of trust and respect needed for open communication and collaboration. Nurses who do not fear reprisal from leadership and perceive a culture of trust will have opportunities to make these changes.

McNaron[40] described characteristics of transformational leaders as those inspiring staff and facilitating cultures of learning. Transformational leaders motivate staff to be more engaged in their practice and to focus on delivery of quality patient-centered care. These leaders demonstrate willingness to review their practice and related patient outcomes and to investigate new technologies and best practices, to ensure they maintain the highest standards of practice.

In the absence of such leaders, McNaron[40] identified strategies that units can adopt to "transform" their learning culture. Examples of these strategies include creation of peer discussion groups, reflective journaling, and activities focused on analysis and validation. An essential element for any strategy was that it resulted in constant examination of current practices for all members of the unit.

Another effective strategy that can foster a unit's growth as a learning practice community is the creation of a "discovery group."[41,42] Discovery groups can be established when nurses identify a research question that is linked to patient-centered care in their unit. Nurses are guided by a faculty mentor from a local nursing school to

---

Box 1
Items from the Support subscales of the modified-LPI consistent with focus group comments

The information I get to do my job is usually accurate

I get enough information to do my job well

Data and information our unit needs are openly shared

I receive information I need at the time I need it to do my job well

Our unit systematically reviews its performance against clearly defined objectives

Senior nurses in our unit support change and development

Regardless of any formal hierarchy in our unit we collaborate and respect each other

Training and development that meet my nursing needs are available

develop a research question, design research, administer an intervention, collect and analyze data, and interpret findings. During weekly sessions, group members review literature, and determine the best methodological approach to answer their research question. Members of discovery groups report increased confidence in their ability to understand research literature, engage in research-related behaviors, and apply research findings to their practice.

How to Begin: Assessing Perioperative Units

Nurses must understand that the first step in the journey to become a learning practice community is a comprehensive assessment of the unit. Detailed examination about perceptions of the unit as a learning culture can guide next steps to plan, implement, and evaluate interventions to strengthen current practices and promote shared goals.

A useful early strategy is to administer an instrument, such as the LPI, to unit leaders and staff to gauge the perceptions of all practitioners about current practices and norms. Baseline data must then be shared with all unit members to identify shared priorities and develop an action plan. Chosen interventions can then be evaluated through comparisons with baseline data and to appropriate patient outcomes. To enable the LPI to be a "living" instrument, unit leaders and staff may also choose to include or remove items that assess current or future learning goals.

Developing Perioperative Environments that Support Learning Opportunities

Rushmer and colleagues,[29–31] whose research focused on a learning practice in primary care settings, provided a framework that could be applied to nursing. According to Rushmer and colleagues,[29–31] primary care settings or clinical nursing units that perform as learning practice communities share a number of critical characteristics. In general, these characteristics include flow of information, staff participation, limited layers of hierarchy, and shared understanding of members' roles. Unit nurses collaborate to establish policies, procedures, councils, and practices. Specialized staff skills, coaching, and reciprocity agreements are shared with other clinical units to proliferate the emergence of systematic learning.

Incentives and rewards for learning are given to staff through praise and recognition of positive practice outcomes. These practice outcomes are then permanently recorded within the clinical unit so that key skills and decisions are maintained in the unit's history. Financial support for research and development programs is a high priority and funding is made available even when constraints exist.

Finally, a clinical unit that is a strong learning practice fosters interactions and relationships based on mutual respect and trust. Collective learning leads to shared investment in developed ideas and implementation of best practices that meet unit needs. For each practicing nurse, learning becomes an issue of engaging in and contributing to the practices in their clinical nursing unit. For the clinical nursing unit, it means that learning is an issue of refining best practices and ensuring new generations of nurses are taught this practice.[41] Collective learning is not just a simple summation of all individual learning, but rather the synergy of shared learning experiences and efforts. The more knowledgeable and capable a team becomes, the more innovative it will be in providing care for patients.[29–31] Advocating for learning practice communities within your perioperative environment is a means to promote positive quality care and nurse outcomes.

REFERENCES

1. McGee P. Perioperative nursing: a review of the literature. Br J Theatre Nurs 1991; 1:12–7.

2. Gruendemann BJ, Fernsebner B. Comprehensive perioperative nursing. Boston: Jones & Bartlett; 1995.
3. Newland CE. The joys of perioperative nursing. Can Oper Room Nurs J 2007; 25(2):20, 22, 23, 25-8.
4. Mackintosh C. Making patients better: a qualitative descriptive study of registered nurses' reasons for working in surgical areas. J Clin Nurs 2007;16(6):1134-40.
5. AORN. Nursing Research. 2012. Available at: http://www.aorn.org/Clinical_Practice/Nursing_Research/Nursing_Research.aspx#axzz209QvNIXB. Accessed July 9, 2012.
6. Robinson M, Cottrell D. Health professionals in multi-disciplinary and multi-agency teams: changing professional practice. J Interprof Care 2005;19(6):547-60.
7. Nelson C, Batalden P, Godrey M. Quality by design. San Francisco (CA): Jossey-Bass; 2007.
8. Norton EK, Martin C, Micheli AJ. Patients count on it: an initiative to reduce incorrect counts and prevent retained surgical items. AORN J 2012;95(1):109-21.
9. Tucker AL, Singer SJ, Hayes JE, et al. Front-line staff perspectives on opportunities for improving the safety and efficiency of hospital work systems. Health Serv Res 2008;43(5 Pt 2):1807-29.
10. Armstrong K, Laschinger HK, Wong C. Workplace empowerment and magnet hospital characteristics as predictors of patient safety climate. J Nurs Care Qual 2009;24(1):55-62.
11. Donahue L, Rader S, Triolo PK. Nurturing innovation in the critical care environment: transforming care at the bedside. Crit Care Nurs Clin North Am 2008; 20(4):465-9.
12. Koll B, Straub T, Jalon H, et al. The CLABs collaborative: a regionwide effort to improve the quality of care in hospitals. Jt Comm J Qual Patient Saf 2008; 34(12):713-23.
13. Fung-Kee-Fung M, Goubanova E, Sequeira K, et al. Development of communities of practice to facilitate quality improvement initiatives in surgical oncology. Qual Manag Health Care 2008;17(2):174-85.
14. Parsons ML, Clark P, Marshall M, et al. Team behavioral norms: a shared vision for a healthy patient care workplace. Crit Care Nurs Q 2007;30(3):213-8.
15. Parsons ML, Newcomb M. Developing a healthy OR workplace. AORN J 2007; 85(6):1213-4.
16. IOM. Keeping patients safe: transforming the work environment of nurses. Washington, DC: National Academies Press; 2004.
17. Cvetic E. Communication in the perioperative setting. AORN J 2011;94(3):261-70.
18. Gillespie BM, Chaboyer W, Wallis M, et al. Resilience in the operating room: developing and testing of a resilience model. J Adv Nurs 2007;59(4):427-38.
19. Knol J, van Linge R. Innovative behaviour: the effect of structural and psychological empowerment on nurses. J Adv Nurs 2009;65(2):359-70.
20. IOM. Future of nursing: leading change, advancing health. Washington, DC: National Academies Press; 2010.
21. Singer SJ, Rosen A, Zhao S, et al. Comparing safety climate in naval aviation and hospitals: implications for improving patient safety. Health Care Manage Rev 2010;35(2):134-46.
22. Garvin D, Edmondson AC, Gino F. Is yours a learning organization? Harv Bus Rev 2008;86(3):109-16.
23. Sexton JB, Makary MA, Tersigni AR, et al. Teamwork in the operating room: front-line perspectives among hospitals and operating room personnel. Anesthesiology 2006;105(5):877-84.

24. Reason JT, Carthey J, de Leval MR. Diagnosing "vulnerable system syndrome": an essential prerequisite to effective risk management. Qual Health Care 2001; 10(Suppl 2):ii21–5.
25. Celik J. Decreasing preoperative delays—a rapid process improvement project. AORN J 2003;77(4):737–41.
26. Prowse MA, Heath V. Working collaboratively in health care contexts: the influence of bioscientific knowledge on patient outcomes. Nurse Educ Today 2005; 25(2):132–9.
27. Espin S, Lingard L, Baker GR, et al. Persistence of unsafe practice in everyday work: an exploration of organizational and psychological factors constraining safety in the operating room. Qual Saf Health Care 2006;15(3):165–70.
28. Tucker AL, Edmondson AC. Why hospitals don't learn from failures: organizational and psychological dynamics that inhibit system change. Calif Manag Rev 2003;45(2):55–72.
29. Rushmer R, Kelly D, Lough M, et al. Introducing the learning practice—I. The characteristics of learning organizations in primary care. J Eval Clin Pract 2004;10(3):375–86.
30. Rushmer R, Kelly D, Lough M, et al. Introducing the learning practice—II. Becoming a learning practice. J Eval Clin Pract 2004;10(3):387–98.
31. Rushmer R, Kelly D, Lough M, et al. Introducing the learning practice—III. Leadership, empowerment, protected time and reflective practice as core contextual conditions. J Eval Clin Pract 2004;10(3):399–405.
32. Li LC, Grimshaw JM, Nielsen C, et al. Use of communities of practice in business and health care sectors: a systematic review. Implement Sci 2009;4:27.
33. Rushmer RK, Parker J, Phillips S. Introducing self-directed primary care teams in the NHS: an overview of initial strategic issues. In: Rushmer RK, Davies HTO, Tavakoli MT, et al, editors. Organisation Development in Health Care: Strategic Issues in Health Care Management. Ashgate, Aldershot: Gower; 2002. p. 51–9.
34. Lave J, Wenger E. Situated learning: legitimate peripheral participation. Cambridge (United Kingdom): Cambridge University Press; 1991.
35. Rushmer R, Kelly D, Lough M, et al. The learning practice inventory: diagnosing and developing learning practices in the UK. J Eval Clin Pract 2007;13(2):206–11.
36. Swenson-Britt E. Clinical nursing units as learning practice communities: Relations between research self-collective efficacy and quality of care and nurse outcomes [dissertation]. San Antonio (TX): Nursing, University of Texas Health Science Center at San Antonio; 2011.
37. Swenson-Britt E, Berndt A. Development and psychometric testing of the Nurses Research Self-Efficacy Scale: NURSES. J Nurs Meas 2012;21(1), in press.
38. Lake ET. Development of the practice environment scale of the nursing work index. Res Nurs Health 2002;25(3):176–88.
39. Lake ET. The nursing practice environment: measurement and evidence. Med Care Res Rev 2007;64(Suppl 2):104S–22S.
40. McNaron ME. Using transformational learning principles to change behavior in the OR. AORN J 2009;89(5):851–60.
41. Swenson-Britt E, Reineck C. Research education for clinical nurses: a pilot study to determine research self-efficacy in critical care nurses. J Contin Educ Nurs 2009;40(10):1–9.
42. Wenger E, McDermott R, Snyder WM. Cultivating communities of practice. Boston: Harvard Business School Press; 2002.

Advocating for Perioperative Nursing and Patient Safety

Donna A. Ford, MSN, RN-BC, CNOR

KEYWORDS

- Advocacy • Perioperative nursing • Practice resources

KEY POINTS

- Professional nursing associations provide support through practice resources, education, and legislative activities.
- Advocacy between perioperative nurses and professional nursing associations is symbiotic, and ultimately serves to further improve the quality of patient care and the profession of nursing.

INTRODUCTION

Advocacy is the foundation of nursing practice. Nurses have the opportunity to act as a patient advocate in every patient encounter by focusing on the patient's specific wishes and by ensuring that care is provided in the safest manner possible.[1] The dictionary defines an advocate as "one that supports or promotes the interests of another."[2] Advocating for patients includes speaking up to ensure safe and effective care and supporting a patient's right to make health care choices.[3] Nurses also advocate for patients collectively, for each other, and for the nursing profession.

Perioperative nurses have a unique patient population. The nurse has only a small window of time to interact with surgical patients before they are sedated or anesthetized. In addition to his or her expertise in the perioperative arena, the nurse bases his or her advocacy efforts on the information gathered from the patient and family, other professionals, and the patient's chart to advocate successfully. In addition, however, the Association of periOperative Registered Nurses (AORN) provides a wealth of resources to empower the perioperative nurse to advocate successfully for surgical patients. Belonging to one's professional nursing organization can be an excellent support system for advocating for patients and the nursing profession.

Professional associations have members, and through these members the professional nursing associations then establish "a code of ethics, standards of care and practice, and policies that govern the profession."[4]

Department of Nursing, College of Medicine, Mayo Clinic, 200 First Street SW, Rochester, MN 55905, USA
E-mail address: ford.donna@mayo.edu

Perioperative Nursing Clinics 7 (2012) 425–432
http://dx.doi.org/10.1016/j.cpen.2012.08.007
1556-7931/12/$ – see front matter © 2012 Elsevier Inc. All rights reserved.
periopnursing.theclinics.com

Through a professional organization, members have the ability to participate actively in personal and professional growth and development through educational and practice requirements, educational activities, research, committee participation, leadership opportunities, and participating in the governance of the organization by being actively involved in decision making at the House of Delegates. The organization facilitates patient advocacy through a code of ethics, standards of practice, position statements, practice tool kits, education, and networking. A professional organization is a strong advocate when it brings the voices of all of its members to the table when soliciting improvements in the advocacy environment for patients and nurses.

ADVOCATING FOR PATIENTS THROUGH PROFESSIONAL NURSING ASSOCIATION MEMBERSHIP

Nursing is a profession built on trust. Nurses are granted a license to practice by their licensing body and the public trusts nurses to provide quality care. Three "foundational" American Nurses Association (ANA) publications detail the practice environment for nurses: *The Code of Ethics for Nurses with Interpretative Statements*, *The Social Policy Statement: Essence of the Profession*, and *Nursing: Scope and Standards of Practice*. All 3 documents address the advocacy role of both professional nursing associations and individual nurses.[5] For instance, Provision 3 of the Code of Ethics for Nurses states "The nurse promotes, advocates for, and strives to protect the health, safety, and rights of the patient."[4]

A licensed registered nurse is granted legal authority as an individual to practice nursing. According to Beyea, this "authority implies that nurses have a significant responsibility to act in the best interests of the patients in their care."[6] As one of the professions most trusted by the public, nurses are responsible for providing the best care possible. This delivery of care requires both academic and continuing education and practice according to evidence-based recommendations. Furthermore, "all nurses are responsible for practicing in accordance with recognized standards of professional nursing practice and the recognized professional code of ethics."[4]

Professional associations develop resources to assist nurses keeping current with evidence-based practice, professional issues, and advancing technology. Association members have access to organizations' peer-reviewed professional nursing journals (both print and online), electronic newsletters, and association Web sites. Access to much of the information is restricted to members, making membership in a professional organization a valuable resource for all nurses.

A standardized nursing language facilitates the nurse's ability to advocate for both patients and nursing. Common terminology that nurses use to document assessments, interventions, and outcomes facilitates improved patient care, assessment of nursing competency, comparisons of quality outcomes for nursing interventions, assessment of adherence to standards of practice, and the usefulness of research outcomes.[7,8]

Examples from perioperative nursing demonstrate the link between standardized nursing language patient-care models and advocating for the patient. The Perioperative Nursing Data Set (PNDS), standardized perioperative nursing language, developed by AORN volunteer members and staff, was recognized as specialty nomenclature by the ANA in 1999. The patient is in the center of the Perioperative Patient-Focused Model, indicating the true focus of perioperative nursing care as patient-centric. One PNDS outcome statement declares "the patient is the recipient of competent and ethical care within legal standards of practice." The outcome definition states: "Care providers in the perioperative environment provide health services within their legal and ethical scope of practice. Health care providers are responsible for meeting legal, institutional, professional and regulatory standards." PNDS intervention 730 states that the perioperative nurse "acts as patient advocate by protecting the patient from incompetent, unethical or illegal practices."[9]

ADVOCATING FOR PERIOPERATIVE NURSES THROUGH PROFESSIONAL ASSOCIATION MEMBERSHIP

Nursing professional associations have represented nurses in our society for more than 100 years. The earliest associations were formed as part of the process of establishing nursing as a profession and to ensure competence.[7] Matthews defines a professional association as "an organization of practitioners who judge one another as professionally competent and who have banded together to perform social functions which they cannot perform in their separate capacity as individuals."[5] This "association" is a significant key to the advocacy role provide for nurses by professional associations. A professional nursing association serves as a collective voice of its nurses when addressing social, ethical, or legislative concerns.[3]

Two professional nursing associations represent the interests of all nurses, regardless of specialty. The International Council of Nurses (ICN) is a federation of more than 130 national nursing associations working internationally to ensure quality health care, advancement of nursing knowledge, and a competent and satisfied nursing workforce.[10] The ANA represents the interests of 3.1 million registered nurses in the United States.[11] Individual associations represent the various nursing specialties. The AORN is committed to promoting excellence in perioperative nursing practice, advancing the profession, and supporting the professional perioperative registered nurse.[12]

Regardless of specialty or area of interest, professional nursing associations advocate for nurses by providing clinical practice standards, educational resources, and a code of ethics. Provision 9 of the ANA Code of Ethics for Nurses states: "The profession of nursing, as represented by associations and their members, is responsible for articulating nursing values, for maintaining the integrity of the profession and its practice, and for shaping social policy... Through critical self-reflection and self-evaluation, associations must foster change within themselves, seeking to move the professional community toward its stated ideals."[13]

Although some resources are restricted to members, the ANA, AORN, and many other nursing specialty associations provide public access to a wealth of resources. Professionalism in nursing includes the expectation that nurses will belong to a professional association. The ANA Code of Ethics for Nurses states: "The nurse participates in the advancement of the profession through contributions to practice, education, administration and knowledge development."[14] Professional nursing associations provide resources including evidence-based practice recommendations, patient and health care worker safety tools, peer-reviewed journals, specialty education, and professional networking sites and discussion platforms. Association membership is a bidirectional and multidimensional. Membership dues help to provide the funds and the manpower required to produce these resources, which benefit the members personally and professionally.

HEALTHY WORK ENVIRONMENT

An excellent example of advocacy by professional nursing associations working for the interests of nurses and patients is the development in 2001 of Standards for Establishing and Sustaining Healthy Work Environments by the American Association of Critical-Care Nurses (AACN). These standards represent "evidence-based and relationship-centered principles of professional performance." Developing the standards was followed by developing relevant resources that nurses and hospitals could use to implement these standards.[15]

The publication of *Silence Kills: The Seven Crucial Conversations for Healthcare* in 2005 presented data from a study by VitalSmarts and AACN on communication in health care and its impact on patient safety and job satisfaction. The study results indicated that the majority of health care professionals who witness less than optimal behavior confront their colleagues about their concerns. The study concluded that:

> *The 10% of healthcare workers who confidently raise crucial concerns observe better patient outcomes, work harder, are more satisfied, and are more committed to staying in their jobs. If more healthcare workers could behave like the influential 10%, the result would be significant reductions in medical errors, increased patient safety, higher productivity, and lower turnover.[16]*

In 2010, a follow-up study by VitalSmarts, AACN, and AORN, *The Silent Treatment*, suggest that when it comes to creating healthy work environments that ensure optimal quality of care, individual skills and personal motivation will not be enough to reduce harm and save lives unless speaking up is also supported by the social and structural elements within the organization. Changing entrenched behavior in health care organizations will require a multifaceted approach and, to this end, the investigators provide a series of recommendations that leaders can follow to improve people's ability to hold crucial conversations. The study concluded that while safety tools are one part of the solution to improving patient care, they do not compensate for crucial conversation failures in the hospital. Silence still kills, and the time has come for health care systems to make candor a core competence.[17] These studies are prime examples of professional nursing associations collaborating with other experts to promote advocacy by providing valuable information to educate nurses and the health care environment. Such studies provide excellent resources for nurses at all levels to understand the complexities of teamwork, communication, and patient safety. Addressing communication challenges is essential to establishing a culture of safety.

PERIOPERATIVE NURSES AS ADVOCATES FOR PROFESSIONAL NURSING ASSOCIATIONS

Involvement in professional associations can be a very rewarding experience, both professionally and personally. In addition to supporting the profession as it strives to improve the patient care environment, the personal "return on investment" for active participation includes meeting and learning from colleagues, networking, and opportunities for professional advancement such as writing for publication, giving presentations at meetings and conferences, working on national committees, holding an elective office, and participating in the governance of the organization.

PROFESSIONAL RESPONSIBILITY AND MAINTAINING COMPETENCE

With advances in research and technology, the nursing knowledge base is continually evolving and expanding. Nurses have an ethical and professional responsibility to pursue both academic and continuing education to maintain currency and competency throughout their careers. The ANA Code of Ethics for Nurses (Provision 5) states that "the nurse owes the same duties to self as others, including the responsibility to preserve integrity and safety, to maintain competence and to continue personal and professional growth."[13] Duties also include personal responsibility for assuring competence, continued professional learning, and peer review of performance. Assurance of competence is a shared responsibility of the individual nurse, the nursing profession, professional associations, credentialing and certification group, employers, and regulatory groups.[4] Nurses with "professional commitment," meaning an active involvement in maintaining current clinical knowledge and an awareness of current professional issues, contribute to enhanced patient safety and patient-perceived quality of care.[18]

EVIDENCE-BASED PRACTICE

Reducing the number of errors committed and using evidence-based nursing practices results in higher quality nursing care. The Agency for Healthcare Policy and Research (AHRQ) promotes evidence-based practice in an effort "to improve quality, effectiveness and appropriateness of healthcare" and to assist organizations in this process.[19] Developing practice recommendations through analysis of scientific evidence is a common example. Professional organizations are expected to provide a foundation on which to base recommendations supported by scientific evidence.[20] Evidence-based practice is a hallmark of professional organizations and is described as an "essential method of improving patient care by promoting decisions based on scientific evidence rather than the opinion of an individual health care provider."[19]

Serving on a national committee is an excellent opportunity to participate in advocacy for patients and the nursing profession. For instance, it was a committee of AORN members that selected the method to be used for rating the strength of the scientific evidence for perioperative practice recommendations. Use of evidence-based practice, basing clinical practice decisions on proven scientific evidence, has become the expectation in the nursing profession. Choosing practice option based on "this is the way we have always done it" or "this seems like a good idea" is no longer acceptable.

LIFELONG LEARNING

Competence in nursing requires continuing ones education and pursuing professional development for the duration of one's career. Advances in technology and research, and the increasing complexity of patient care require nurses to seek additional education and training in order to practice safely and effectively. The recent Institute of Medicine Report on the Future of Nursing[21] identifies key points that stressed the importance of education for nurses, including:

- Nurses should practice to the fullest extent of their education and training
- Nurses should achieve higher levels of education and training through an improved education system that promotes seamless academic progression

To be an effective advocate, nurses need to recognize situations in which patients may need an advocate, determine the best interests of the patient, and identify the actions needed to protect those interests.[22] Professional associations often have foundations that support their education initiative. For example, the AORN Foundation funds educational sessions, seminars, and webinars, and provides academic and professional development scholarships. In 2011, the AORN Foundation awarded 288 professional development scholarships totaling $192,000, and has awarded $1.7 million in academic scholarships over the past 20 years. The AORN Foundation also funds research projects and the development of patient safety resources.[23]

SPECIALTY NURSING CERTIFICATION

While the minimum standard for nursing practice is licensure, certification is one way that nurses can develop and demonstrate a higher level of competence.[24] Achieving specialty nursing certification validates experience, specialty knowledge, and clinical judgment, and is an indication of excellence in nursing practice. As a regulated profession, the public has the right to know when nurses have successfully validated their nursing knowledge beyond the minimum standard of licensure. There are benefits to the public, employers, and nurses from nurses who achieve nursing specialty certification. According to the AACN, certification is a step on the path to the "advancement of nursing professionalism, higher standards of care, and better patient outcomes."[25]

The Magnet designation or becoming a designated center of excellence is another indication of advocacy for patients and for nurses. Such facilities strive to create a solid professional practice infrastructure with leadership committed to providing a supportive, autonomous, and empowered practice environment for nurses. This type of practice environment, with highly skilled nurses and responsive systems, is shown to have reduced patient mortality[26] The American Board of Nursing Specialties states that certified nurses contribute to improved quality of patient care and that certification has a positive effect on patient safety and overall patient care. Patients have increasingly complex needs, and the needs of these patients are best met with registered nurses certified in their nursing specialty.[27] A study by Kendall-Gallagher and colleagues[28] correlated nursing specialty certification with inpatient mortality and failure to rescue. One conclusion drawn by these investigators was that nurse specialty certification is associated with better patient outcomes.

There are many ways by which nurses maintain competence, including precepting, mentoring and coaching, creation of educational resources for patients or staff, updating procedural guidelines to include most current evidence-based practice, development of a survey or questionnaire, involvement in quality improvement projects, professional writing, contributions to a professional organization, educational presentations, and teaching academic nursing courses.[23] According to Tomajan,[29] nurses are increasingly positioned to advocate more effectively than ever before not only for patients but also for themselves and the nursing profession.

SUMMARY

Every nurse has the opportunity to advocate for patients, for nurses, and for the profession of nursing. Pursuing lifelong learning and competency leads to patient safety and improved overall patient care. Participating actively in a professional association provides the nurse with resources and opportunities for personal and professional growth. At the same time, members provide the association with resources, both funds and manpower, for advocating on a grander scale. Association membership broadens a nurse's sphere of advocacy and increases the impact one nurse can have on outcomes for patients, nurses, and the nursing profession.

REFERENCES

1. Beyea SC. Patient advocacy—nurses keeping patients safe. AORN J 2005;81(5): 1046–7.
2. Merriam-Webster dictionary. Available at: http://www.merriam-webster.com/dictionary/advocate. Accessed May 30, 2012.

3. Schroeter K. Advocacy in perioperative nursing practice. AORN J 2000;71(6): 1207–20.
4. American Nurses Association. Social context of nursing. In: Carol J. Bickford, Katherine C. Brewer, editors. Nursing's social policy statement-the essence of the profession. Silver Spring (MD): Nursebooks.org; 2010. p. 5–6.
5. Matthews JH. Role of professional organizations in advocating for the nursing profession. Online J Issues Nurs 2012;17(1). Available at: http://www.nursingworld.org/MainMenuCategories/ANAMarketplace/ANAPeriodicals/OJIN/TableofContents/Vol-17-2012/No1-Jan-2012/Professional-Organizations-and-Advocating.html. Accessed May 30, 2012.
6. Beyea SC. Are you just a nurse? AORN J 2008;87(2):441–4.
7. Allen G. Maximizing nurse' advocacy role to improve patient outcomes. AORN J 2000;71(5):1038–49.
8. Rutherford MA. Standardized nursing language: what does it mean for nursing practice? Online J Issues Nurs 2008;13(1):4, 12, 14.
9. Petersen C. Perioperative nursing data set: the perioperative nursing vocabulary. 3rd edition. Denver (CO): AORN, Inc; 2011.
10. International Council of Nurses. About ICN. Available at: http://www.icn.ch/about-icn/about-icn/. Accessed May 31, 2012.
11. American Nurses Association, 2011 ANA annual report. Available at: http://nursingworld.org/FunctionalMenuCategories/AboutANA/2011AnnualReport.html. Accessed June 10, 2012.
12. Association of Perioperative Registered Nurses. In: About AORN. Available at: http://www.aorn.org. Accessed May 31, 2012.
13. American Nurses Association (ANA). Code of ethics for nurses with interpretive statements. Available at: http://www.nursingworld.org/MainMenuCategories/EthicsStandards/CodeofEthicsforNurses/Code-of-Ethics.pdf. Accessed May 30, 2012.
14. IBID.
15. Association of Critical-Care Nurses. AACN standards for establishing and sustaining healthy work environments: a journey to excellence—executive summary. December 2005.
16. VitalSmarts and AACN. Silence kills: the seven crucial conversations for healthcare. Available at: http://www.silenttreatmentstudy.com/silencekills/. Accessed May 31, 2012.
17. VitalSmarts, AACN, and AORN. The Silent Treatment: why safety tools and checklists aren't enough to save lives. 2010. Available at: http://www.silenttreatmentstudy.com/Silent%20Treatment%20Executive%20Summary.pdf and http://www.silenttreatmentstudy.com/. Accessed May 30, 2012.
18. Teng CI, Dai YT, Shyu YI, et al. Professional commitment, patient safety and patient-perceived care quality. J Nurs Scholarsh 2009;41(3):301–9.
19. Agency for Healthcare Quality and Research. In: Evidence-based practice centers. Available at: http://www.ahrq.gov/clinic/epc/. Accessed June 10, 2012.
20. Steelman VM, Pape T, King CA, et al. Selection of a method to rate the strength of scientific evidence for AORN recommendations. AORN J 2011; 93(4):433–43.
21. Commission of the Robert Wood Johnson Foundation Initiative on the Future Of Nursing. The future of nursing: influencing change, advancing health. Washington, DC: National Academies Press; 2011. Available at: http://www.iom.edu/Reports/2010/The-Future-of-Nursing-Leading-Change-Advancing-Health. Accessed June 7, 2012.

22. Bu X, Jezewski MA. Developing a mid-range theory of patient advocacy through concept analysis. J Adv Nurs 2006;57(1):101–10.
23. Byrne M, Schroeter K, Mower J. Perioperative specialty certification: the CNOR as evidence for Magnet Excellence. AORN J 2010;91(5):618–22.
24. Fleischman R, Meyer L, Watson C. Best practices in creating a culture of certification. AACN Adv Crit Care 2011;22:33–49.
25. IBID.
26. Smith AP. Patient advocacy: roles for nurses and leaders. Nurs Econ 2004;22(2): 88–90.
27. American Board of Nursing Specialties (ABNS). A position statement on the value of specialty nursing certification. March 5, 2005. Available at: http://www. nursingcertification.org/resources-position.html. Retrieved June 2, 2012.
28. Kendall-Gallagher D, Aiken LH, Sloane DM, et al. Nurse specialty certification, inpatient mortality, and failure to rescue. J Nurs Scholarsh 2011;43:188–94.
29. Tomajan K. Advocating for nurses and nursing. Online J Issues Nurs 2012;17(1):4.

Advocating through Nursing Specialty Organizations

Amy L. Hader, JD

KEYWORDS

- Advocacy • Nursing specialty organization • Government affairs
- Legislative principles

KEY POINTS

- There are approximately 160,000 nurses practicing in perioperative care in the United States.
- The Association of periOperative Registered Nurses (AORN) advocates for the perioperative nurse.
- AORN establishes practice recommendations and legislative priorities for its 40,000 members and the perioperative nursing field in general.

The Association of periOperative Registered Nurses represents the interests of more than 160,000 perioperative nurses by providing nursing education, standards, and practice resources—including the peer-reviewed, monthly publication AORN Journal—to enable optimal outcomes for patients undergoing operative and other invasive procedures. AORN's 42,000 registered nurse members manage, teach, and practice perioperative nursing, are enrolled in nursing education or are engaged in perioperative research. The AORN Government Affairs Department supports advocacy efforts on behalf of perioperative nurses before legislative and regulatory bodies at both the state and federal levels. Based on recommendations from the association's National Legislative Committee and the President-elect, each year the AORN Board of Directors establishes legislative priorities for the organization. The Government Affairs Department pursues activities in legislative and regulatory arenas nationwide in support of these goals.

In addition to supporting nursing priorities such as workplace safety, whistleblower protection, and safe staffing, AORN's legislative priorities focus specifically on the perioperative priorities of (1) ensuring that each surgical patient has a perioperative registered nurse circulator dedicated to them for the duration of their procedure, and (2) preserving and protecting the perioperative registered nurses' scope of practice, including the role of the registered nurse first assistant (RNFA). AORN also monitors, evaluates and responds to proposed legislative initiatives by allied health care professionals that may affect perioperative nursing and patient safety in the operating room (OR) environment (**Box 1**).

AORN, 2170 South Parker Road, Suite 400, Denver, CO 80231, USA
E-mail address: Ahader@aorn.org

Perioperative Nursing Clinics 7 (2012) 433–436
http://dx.doi.org/10.1016/j.cpen.2012.08.003
periopnursing.theclinics.com
1556-7931/12/$ – see front matter © 2012 Elsevier Inc. All rights reserved.

Box 1
AORN's Principles to be Used in Evaluating Allied Health Legislative Initiatives

AORN's legislative principles are guidelines for reviewing and evaluating legislation related to allied health personnel to protect the safety of the patient and the scope of practice of the perioperative nurse. AORN evaluates and considers lending support to initiatives that meet the following criteria:

1. Evaluation of legislation related to allied health personnel in the perioperative environment will be guided by AORN position statements as approved by the House of Delegates.

2. If the legislated practice of the allied health personnel falls within perioperative nursing practice, as defined by the AORN position statements, the regulation of this practice must be through the state Board of Nursing or the allied health personnel must function under Registered Nurse delegations and be supervised by a registered nurse.

3. The allied health personnel's range of functions must be precisely defined in the legislation. The definition must not be overly broad, and it may not permit the practice of nursing.

4. Legislation that specifies a range of functions for allied health personnel may not prohibit registered nurses from performing the perioperative registered nurse's scope of practice.

5. Statutory regulation of allied health personnel must provide the public with protection of accepted regulatory standards including establishment of an effective mechanism for discipline.

AORN Government Affairs staff work proactively with both paid lobbyists and AORN's perioperative nurse member volunteers to advance and respond to legislative initiatives at the state level. The AORN National Legislative Committee meets monthly by telephone to review current issues and get updated information from AORN. In many states, AORN does not have paid lobbyists and relies exclusively on local perioperative nurse advocates who educate their health care colleagues and the public about the importance of an initiative, attend state lobby days, meet with representatives concerning AORN's position on certain legislation, maintain momentum on grassroots campaigns, and generally stay informed and involved with advocacy issues in the state.

AORN's Government Affairs department urges all perioperative nurses to become advocacy leaders in their states. AORN includes an advocacy section in its weekly e-mail newsletter and Web site tools to facilitate the nurses' efforts to familiarize themselves with AORN's legislative priorities, learn what is happening in their state, and contact their AORN State Coordinator to learn more about current legislative initiatives. AORN members are encouraged to become active with the legislature at the state level. Attending a state lobby day and inviting legislators or legislative candidates to a State Council or AORN chapter meeting are excellent ways of engaging and developing relationships with those who vote on legislation that affects nursing. Perioperative nurse advocates can also invite lawmakers to their hospital, Ambulatory Surgery Center (ASC) or place of employment for an OR tour and offer to be a resource to state legislators and their staff on OR and nursing issues in the state.

AORN is also actively involved in advocating for the profession of nursing. The organization's activities and services are closely aligned with the recommendations of the Institute of Medicine report *Future of Nursing: Leading Change, Advancing Health*. AORN recently joined the Champion Nursing Coalition, a diverse national coalition representing business, consumer and health professional organizations that support the IOM *Future of Nursing*: Campaign for Action. In addition, AORN is a member of many organizations, committees, and task forces that affect the practice of nursing, the care of patients, and the health of our nation.

AORN and the American Nurses Association have observer status at the American Medical Association House of Delegates, where they regularly represent nursing's position on scope of practice barriers. AORN is also a member of the Nursing Community, a forum for national professional nursing associations to build consensus and advocate for nursing practice, education, and research issues. The Nursing Community collaborates to support the education and practice of registered nurses and advance practice nurses, which directly affects the quality, access, and cost of health care and the overall health of our nation. AORN participates on the National Quality Forum and is a founding member of the Ambulatory Surgery Center Quality Collaborative, a group that advocates strongly for sharing reliable quality information with the public to give consumers the opportunity to make informed health care choices.

AORN sits on the American College of Surgeons Committee on Perioperative Care, the American Society of Anesthesiologists Surgical Care Committee, and the Centers for Medicare and Medicaid Services Surgical Care Improvement Project, the Board of Directors of the Nursing Alliance for Quality Care (a pilot project funded by the Robert Wood Johnson Foundation to unify nursing's policy voice to achieve a sustainable impact on the quality of care that the American public receives); and the Industry Partners for Patient Safety, an industry coalition (consisting of industry representatives, regulatory agencies, and health care providers) dedicated to partnering health care professional organizations to promote and support patient safety. In addition, AORN was invited by the World Health Organization (WHO) to participate in the conference held in Geneva, Switzerland to develop the Surgical Safety Checklist. AORN collaborated with Institute for Healthcare Improvement in the spread of the WHO Surgical Checklist. AORN was a founding member of the Council on Surgical and Perioperative Safety. The council has multidisciplinary representatives from many health care professional associations.

AORN's Recommended Practices are developed in collaboration with liaisons from the American Association of Nurse Anesthetists, the American College of Surgeons, the American Society of Anesthesiologists, the Association for Professionals in Infection Control and Epidemiology, the Centers for Disease Control and Prevention, and the International Association of Healthcare Central Service Material Management. AORN recently implemented an evidence ranking system for its Recommended Practices. The system allows the Recommended Practices to be recognized by the National Guideline Clearing house, a public resource for evidence-based clinical practice guidelines.

AORN also offers continuing education activities through: face-to-face meetings, Webinars, *AORN Journal*, certificate program for ambulatory surgery managers, tool kits, and an annual Leadership Academy for chapter officers and other interested members. One of these activities, the Confidence-Based Learning Modules for Perioperative Nurses, is a cutting-edge educational program designed to test the participants' level of knowledge and level of confidence in that knowledge, allowing the learner to repeat the education until they have achieved mastery of the knowledge. Many AORN offerings and activities incorporate information on the need for constant advocacy on behalf of perioperative nursing practice and the nursing profession's constant contributions to improving patient safety.

RESOURCES

Association of periOperative Registered Nurses http://www.aorn.org/.
American Medical Association House of Delegates http://www.ama-assn.org/ama/
   pub/about-ama/our.../house-delegates.page.

National Quality Forum http://www.qualityforum.org/.

Ambulatory Surgery Center Quality Collaborative http://www.ascquality.org/.

American College of Surgeons Committee on Perioperative Care http://www.facs.org/about/committees/cpc/index.html.

American Society of Anesthesiologists Surgical Care Committee http://www.asahq.org/For-Members/About-ASA/ASA-Committees.aspx.

Centers for Medicare and Medicaid Services Surgical Care Improvement Project http://www.cms.gov/.

Council on Surgical and Perioperative Safety http://www.cspsteam.org/.

Advocating for the New Perioperative Nurse

Tiffany Facile, BS, RN, CNOR

KEYWORDS

- Nursing • Perioperative setting • Orientation • Bullying

KEY POINTS

- Collaboration is needed with local nursing programs to facilitate their efforts to include perioperative nursing in their curricula.
- New nurses must be welcomed into the operating room and their success as perioperative team members facilitated.
- Professionals need to support every member of their surgical teams, embrace process changes, learn from failures, and celebrate successes.

INTRODUCTION

There is more than an element of truth in the saying that nurses eat their young. Have you ever been made to feel inadequate by a colleague? Has a colleague ever embarrassed you in front of other team members? Have you ever purposely sabotaged a coworker or caused one to look bad? These questions are uncomfortable and disturbing to answer, but they address a real and destructive dynamic in nursing, including within the perioperative setting.

The operating room (OR) is a stressful environment in which perioperative nurses strive to provide safe patient care under challenging conditions. Patients in the OR are at their most vulnerable, and there is little room for error. New graduates or novice nurses comprise the largest market of available nurses in the United States,[1] and new graduate nurses represent an increasing proportion of nursing staff in hospitals.[2] This group also represents the future of the perioperative workforce.

Orientation to perioperative nursing is necessarily extensive. There is a lot to learn in the perioperative setting (eg, instrumentation, surgical procedures, and protocols) before a nurse can independently provide safe patient care. The more surgical specialties there are, the more complex the orientation. Perioperative orientation is even more challenging because most nursing curricula provide only limited exposure to the surgical setting; clinical rotations through a perioperative department are narrow, and

Avera McKennan Hospital, 1325 South Cliff Avenue, PO Box 5045, Sioux Falls, SD 57117-5045, USA
E-mail address: tiffany.facile@avera.org

Perioperative Nursing Clinics 7 (2012) 437–440
http://dx.doi.org/10.1016/j.cpen.2012.08.012
1556-7931/12/$ – see front matter © 2012 Elsevier Inc. All rights reserved.

usually lack a definitive preceptor.[3] A robust, tenured perioperative nursing workforce depends on the consistent and successful orientation of new perioperative nurses.

Because few graduate nurses are choosing the OR, the perioperative workforce is aging. Most seasoned OR personnel have strong personalities, and the atmosphere is competitive. Too often, the stressful environment can provoke a professional to abandon acceptable behavior, and become openly or passively aggressive. The target of abuse is usually a new employee or one who is not expected to fight back. Young nurses are less likely to complete orientation and join the perioperative workforce in an environment in which there is abuse.

MY STORY

I started my nursing career in a small, community hospital, located in my hometown. As a newly graduated registered nurse, I was energetic, frightened, excited, naive, and motivated to learn everything about health care. In a 25-bed facility, I worked in the emergency room, labor and delivery, coronary care, on medical-surgical units, and in a pediatric area. I valued the experience, grew attached to every area I worked in, and assisted wherever I was needed. I remember working nearly 60-hour weeks when staffing was limited. My education beyond nursing school included basic cardiac courses, trauma nursing core course (TNCC), advanced cardiac life support (ACLS), neonatal resuscitation program (NRP), basic life support (BLS), and I was working on my pediatric advanced life support (PALS).

Although I thoroughly enjoyed the opportunities that this facility offered me, I left my position before the end of my first year because of overbearing, deceitful, and condescending nurse coworkers. For instance, I often discovered that my intravenous fluids and oxygen flow rates would mysteriously vary throughout the day. I heard from other nurses that this was a common thing for the tenured nurses to do. I am not sure whether they were trying to keep me on my toes or promote my failure. Either way, the behavior was unacceptable. It was also well known that the newer nurses were assigned the most challenging patients. The older nurses insisted that this practice was designed to see whether I could handle the nursing profession. However, they offered no help or support when I needed it. I took my concerns to my director who insisted that my accusations were fabricated and unreasonable. Without the support of my colleagues or management, I thought that there was no way that I could learn or succeed.

Having particularly enjoyed the emergency room and coronary care unit, I decided to pursue critical care as my nursing specialty. I relocated to a larger city, and took a position as an intensive care unit (ICU) nurse. In retrospect, I was naive to think that I was well prepared for critical care. I worked mostly night shifts and every other weekend. I had no consistent mentor or preceptor and was given only a brief, 2-month orientation. Although I studied each night about Swan catheters, sepsis, trauma, and cardiac disorders, I knew nothing about giving intravenous dopamine as a titrated infusion while adding dobutamine for severe hypotension, and obtaining blood through an arterial line, not to mention not understanding a pulse pressure. After 6 months of extreme stress and inadequate training, I decided to look for another nursing position. I left the ICU and was hired as a surgical nurse in a clinic setting. This humbling transition brought me to my current position as a clinical nurse educator in a perioperative setting.

Here I have the opportunity to train newly graduated nurses into the perioperative setting. Watching energetic and optimistic nurses blossom into independent practitioners provides me unending satisfaction. However, a few of my orientees have left the OR because of bullying: verbal abuse, passive-aggressive behavior, and unsatisfactory training from preceptors. Experienced nurses have laughed and censured the newer nurses for asking questions and ridiculed their technique; they even criticized the food they ate. Even though there are many more professional nurses than bullies, the negative impact of the few can be devastating.

Although the environment here is generally supportive, I too have been demeaned and demoralized by tenured staff. I have never been a circulator in this hospital, although I am well read and have excellent preceptors. The success of the orientees for whom I am responsible has earned me the respect and support of most of my colleagues. However, while I was studying for the CNOR examination, a colleague disdainfully said to me, "I don't know how you can possibly expect to pass the CNOR examination. You've never functioned as a circulating nurse in a real OR." Her disparaging comment would have made me question my potential for success and the wisdom of pursuing certification had it not been for the enthusiasm and encouragement of others who appreciate my practice.

New nurses must develop confidence in themselves to function in a high-stress environment like the OR. They must have trustworthy mentors and preceptors who bolster their clinical skills and facilitate their social integration into the environment. Competent preceptors provide constructive feedback and encouragement to the new employee who wants to become a competent perioperative nurse and a comfortable member of the OR team. I have noted that the younger nurses absorb new information at a faster rate, want very much to establish positive relationships, and adjust well when the environment welcomes them and provides for their learning needs.

Thanks to my younger nurse colleagues, I have now discovered the value of work/life balance; I no longer work 60-hour weeks. The younger generations, although highly scrutinized and misunderstood, recognize the importance of career commitments but also appreciate their obligations to the other important things in their lives. This balanced viewpoint creates conflict with staff who assume that all good nurses should put their nursing commitments first.

Another source of strife among the generations in nursing is the tenured nurses' belief that, because they learned the hard way, the younger nurses should face the same challenges. I have heard comments such as, "I refuse to make it easy for them. You learn from your mistakes." "I never got an orientation, so why should they?" "They will never learn if they aren't challenged." Overall, this nonprogressive and passive-aggressive behavior creates staff dissatisfaction, increases staff-turnover rate, and can result in negative patient outcomes.

I would like to change how people perceive the perioperative department, and end the negative behaviors and attitudes. I would like nursing schools to extend their programs to include meaningful exposure to the perioperative setting. Surgeons should gladly offer explanations for their quirky demands and strange requests. Health care managers and experienced perioperative nurses should know intuitively that working a 12-hour shift and being on call for the remainder 12 hours, after completing a 24-hour weekend shift, is unacceptable and inappropriate. This demanding work arrangement does not represent a good work ethic or build good nurses.

I realize that change in my workplace starts with me. I know that managing a health care environment is challenging, that financial and human resources are scarce, and that the workforce represents different personalities, different levels of competence, and different individual needs. It takes lots of people to make significant changes, but often that change begins with the efforts of 1 person. When you see the need for change, instead of complaining, share your enthusiasm and ideas with your colleagues and build support for a better way to manage the situation. The Harvard Business School teaches students to bring solutions, not problems. It is more likely that a manager will respond positively to a request to evaluate a potential solution to a problem than to hearing a complaint with no carefully crafted suggestion for improvement.

Another difference in perspective that can promote success in the workplace is the emotionally intelligent work environment that recognizes that individuals have both strengths and weaknesses. Managers in these environments cultivate the strengths of their employees rather than the traditional approach of taking strengths for granted and working on the weaknesses. It is not necessary to be good at everything if you can excel at something your work environment values. The personality that excels in a fast-paced environment with multiple procedures in a short period of time might not be the best for procedures that take many hours and require infinite patience. They form teams of individuals who, collectively, have the best skills for the task at hand. Skilled practitioners do not necessarily make good teachers, and the best practitioners are often terrible managers.

SUMMARY

The current and future generations of nurses will replace the aging perioperative workforce. There must be collaborate with local nursing programs to facilitate efforts to include perioperative nursing in the curricula. New nurses must be welcomed into the OR and their success as perioperative team members facilitated. Old habits, strong personalities, and unprofessional bullying must not occur without opposition. Professionals need to support every member of surgical teams, embrace process changes, learn from failures, and celebrate successes. A concerted effort must be made to change so-called eating-our-young behaviors into practices that empower our young. After all, they will be taking care of us some day.

REFERENCES

1. Friedman MI, Cooper AH, Click E, et al. Specialized new graduate RN critical care orientation: retention and financial impact. Nurs Econ 2011;29(1):7–14.
2. Bratt MM, Felzer HM. Perceptions of professional practice and work environment of new graduates in a nurse residency program. J Contin Educ Nurs 2011;42(12): 559–68. http://dx.doi.org/10.3928/00220124-20110516-03.
3. Lydon C, Burke E. Students experiences of theatre allocations. J Perioper Pract 2012;22(2):45–9.

Advocating for Specific Patient Populations

The Nurse's Nurse
Peer Advocacy in an Alternative Program for Nurses

Michael Van Doren, MSN, RN, CARN

KEYWORDS

- Peer assistance • Nurse advocacy • Colleagues • Alternative programs
- Substance use disorder

KEY POINTS

- Alternative programs for nurses, sometimes known as peer assistance programs, are designed to promote identification of nurses whose practice may be impaired by substance use disorders (SUSs: ie, abuse or dependency on drugs or alcohol) and possibly psychiatric disorders.
- Alternative programs for nurses facilitate preservation of a nursing license and return to work for nurses with SUD who are in recovery.
- A peer assistance advocate is a trained and approved nurse who volunteers to provide one-to-one support for nurses participating in a program.
- Peer assistance advocates provide education to nursing colleagues and employers of program participants.

INTRODUCTION

… sometimes our ordinary labor, administered in the right dose at the right time, can provide extraordinary mercy. And in our world, our colleagues never have to fear facing their darkest hours alone.[1]

Although nurse advocacy is most often associated with stepping up to protect the welfare of a patient or patient population, nurses can also advocate for nurses. Some of our nursing colleagues may have, or may be suspected of having, a substance use disorder (SUD) or psychiatric problem that could impair their ability to provide appropriate patient care. Often these nurses are ignored until there is patient safety incident or near miss that could result in loss of their license to practice and all of the miseries associated with such a traumatic experience.

Provision 3.6 of the American Nurses Association (ANA) Code of Ethics[2] and the ANA's position paper of 2002, "The Profession's Response to the Problem of Addictions and Psychiatric Disorders in Nursing,"[3] address this issue, at least on an ethical and policy level. Well-administered state peer assistance programs can address this

Texas Peer Assistance Program for Nurses, 2200 Kimra Lane, Cedar Park, TX 78613, USA
E-mail address: mvandoren@texasnurses.org

Perioperative Nursing Clinics 7 (2012) 441–446
http://dx.doi.org/10.1016/j.cpen.2012.08.011 **periopnursing.theclinics.com**

situation and facilitate positive outcomes if the nursing professionals are willing to be accountable and participate responsibly in their recovery process.

For more than 25 years, the Texas Peer Assistance Program for Nurses (TPAPN) has operated as the approved peer assistance program for the Texas Board of Nursing. Over the years, TPAPN has grown steadily, saving 1 nurse at a time from what, for many nurses with active SUD or psychiatric disorder, had become a world of despair, darkness, and isolation. Often their peers were not aware of the problem and may have seen nothing untoward with their practice as professional nurses. A cadre of volunteer nurse advocates provides the grace and humanity necessary to advocate for these colleagues. This article provides a general, as well as a detailed, discussion of the advocacy that TPAPN and other alternative programs can provide.

The National Council of State Boards of Nursing (NCSBN) defines an alternative program as "a voluntary, non-public and non-disciplinary program, which offers nurses who meet specified criteria an opportunity to maintain licensure and practice as an alternative to traditional discipline authorized in statute and rule by nursing or other regulatory boards."[4] TPAPN is an alternative peer assistance program of a professional association that collaborates with the Board of Nursing. It is one of the 6 types of alternative programs identified by the NCSBN (2011) that promote the identification, treatment, and monitored reentry to practice of nurses with SUDs.

Alternative programs for nurses in the United States began to proliferate in the late 1970s; currently there are only 9 states without such programs. TPAPN is administered by the Texas Nurses Foundation, the 501(c)(3) charitable, educational, and research arm of the Texas Nurses Association. Since its inception in 1985, TPAPN has distinguished itself among alternative programs for its commitment to and success with advocacy for nurses with active SUD. Participation requirements are stringent, but the success rate for participants is high; TPAPN's internal data reveals that at least 75% of all RNs who return to nursing practice complete the programs successfully (**Box 1**). However, it is TPAPN's volunteer peer advocacy component that distinguishes the program from most alternative programs. TPAPN now has more than 230 active advocates from all levels of nursing and from every part of Texas.

Box 1
Standard requirements of participants in alternative programs

1. Obtain assessment to further ensure their eligibility

2. Sign required program paperwork, including consents

3. Complete recommended treatment

4. Register for and determine random drug testing status, as appropriate, on a daily basis

5. Obtain approval for reentry to nursing practice

6. Adhere to practice restrictions

7. Show safe nursing practice for a minimum of 1 year

8. Document ongoing attendance at self-help meetings (eg, Alcoholics Anonymous and Narcotics Anonymous), along with attendance at facilitated support groups and individual (psychiatric) therapy as warranted

9. Document all prescribed and over-the-counter medications (ongoing)

10. Submit routine self-reports (ongoing)

11. Adhere to program requirements for the period necessary for successful completion (for most alternative programs, this is a minimum of 3 years)

ADVOCACY FOR NURSES: ORGANIZATIONAL/POLICY

TPAPN, whose slogan is "Nurses helping nurses," is a superb example of nurses advocating for their nurse colleagues. The Texas legislature supports peer assistance for nurses by granting administrative authority, funding, referral, confidentiality, and civil immunity through legal statute and reporting provisions under the state's Nurse Practice Act. Although nurses have a great deal of support available at the state level, they often do not experience that same level of support from their peers in the workplace. Too often, nurses have been accused, metaphorically, of eating their young, as well as each other.[5] TPAPN has identified that as many as 50% of nurses referred to the program were terminated without having been referred for professional help, or to TPAPN, or reported to the Board of Nursing. Nurses who have completed the TPAPN program also face this negativity when they seek to return to the workplace.

TPAPN's commitment to nurses helping nurses, in addition to serving as nurse advocates, is to serve as local ambassadors to promote a culture that is life affirming and nurturing but with measured expectations. This positive mission helps TPAPN attract more and more Texas nurses to an advocacy role each year, in which they invest their time and energy to facilitate positive, personal change. Even though the role of peer advocate is not always easy, predictable, or upbeat, TPAPN's nurse advocates think that the positive outcomes outweigh the sacrifices.

ADVOCACY FOR NURSES: INDIVIDUAL

In TPAPN's experience, there are 4 primary groups who serve as nurse advocates. The largest and typically the most enthusiastic group comprises nurses who are in recovery. These nurses usually think that advocating for TPAPN participants helps to strengthen their own recovery. They know firsthand what a lifesaver, and license saver, a peer assistance program can be; how it guides a nurse along a monitored, rehabilitative path. For this group of nurses, volunteering provides a means for giving back, facilitating for others the freedom and joy they have experienced with recovery.

The second group includes nurses who have developed empathy through involvement with colleagues or family members with SUDs or psychiatric disorders. A third group comprises nurse who are seeking professional advancement through service to the profession. Some nurses discover the opportunity when they are looking for contact hour opportunities; nurses can earn contact hours for advocate training workshops. The last group includes nurses who have read articles on peer assistance, have heard about the opportunity through friends, or have attended educational activities and have been inspired to volunteer.

TPAPN advocates often say that just being present, one professional nurse lending support to another, can make an important difference for their participants. It is common for participants to think that they are the only nurses to have ever have sunk so low or have done such bad things. Recovery is a difficult process. Participants must deal with the rigors of TPAPN requirements, must learn to cope positively with their problem, often having to deal simultaneously with the stigma associated with nurses with SUDs and psychiatric disorders.

Nurses come to volunteer with TPAPN for many reasons, sometimes not fully known to themselves, except perhaps the simple desire to help another nurse or to make a difference for the profession 1 nurse at a time. Although the previous personal examples show how advocacy translates between individual nurses, there are many other aspects to the advocacy role. A few salient examples of how peer advocacy may manifest itself are presented later.

Other ways in which nurse advocates participate include facilitating and interpreting the administrative processes for a participant especially during the fog of early recovery.

They communicate regularly with the participant to decrease the feeling of isolation. Advocates visit the participant's colleagues in the workplace to provide support and to explain how the program works, including the rationale and benefits of practice restrictions, and help to identify resources and support groups in the participant's local community. Celebrating the participant's successful completion of the program and envisioning an ongoing personal program of recovery is another form of advocacy. By doing so, they may inspire new graduates to become advocates. Because advocates visit workplaces with their participants, they are also able to identify the facilities and hospitals most willing to hire TPAPN nurses. TPAPN refers to these employers as its partners in recovery.

Maintaining healthy boundaries in the advocate/participant relationship helps advocates identify signs of actual or impending relapse, such as slurred speech, boisterous or unrealistic talk or actions, or failing to follow through with calls or appointments as scheduled. If the participant is noncompliant, has a positive drug test, or is otherwise unsuccessful in completing the program, the advocate may still be able to give support and assistance, helping the nurse to understand available options.

A story worth telling

My preceptorship as a newly graduated registered nurse (RN) was brutal. Still stinging from my first weeks of work, I received a copy of the Texas Board of Nursing newsletter. At the bottom of the page was an advertisement that said, "Nurses helping nurses." That sounded, to me, like a novel idea. Off to Austin I went for advocate training. I came home from that trip with the name of my first participant in my purse.

In the years that followed, I have had largely pleasant experiences as an advocate. There have been many more successes than failures. Being an advocate is rewarding and interesting. However, it is also time consuming. There came a point when I was not the only advocate in my area. One of my participants was now an advocate. Even better, one of her participants completed the program, and also became an advocate. As my priorities shifted, I became less interested in serving as an advocate. Shortly after this decision, I was reminded of the importance of the program.

My 16-year-old son asked to bring a girl to an important family event. It was obviously important to him, and I consented. I knew the authors were in trouble by the time the authors got to the restaurant. She was beautiful and charming, and my son was obviously smitten. I began to ask about her future plans. College? Career planning? The girl sitting beside my precious boy told me that she was going to be a nurse. A nurse? She did not look like a nurse. Not to me.

So I asked her why she wanted to be a nurse. "My mom is a nurse," she replied. "My mom is a nurse, and she is my hero." She described how her mother had always come through for her family. She worked long hours taking care of people, then came home to take care of her children. I told this lovely young lady that I was a nurse as well, and asked for her mother's name. She told me her name, and time stood very still. I knew her mother. I first saw her name on the piece of paper I tucked into my purse in Austin many years ago. Her mother, her hero, was my first participant as an advocate.

At the time, she did not look like a hero. She was late to our meeting at a local coffee shop. She was obviously emotional, and just completing the paperwork was a chore. I remember her doing better, getting it together, calling me less frequently. She completed the program and we lost touch.

I know I do not get credit for her sobriety. She had a program, a sponsor, a case manager, and a support system. I just helped a little with the structure. In this true success story, though, even helping in a small way was an honor. After meeting her daughter, I made it to the next advocate workshop.

Adapted from Butcher-Ortiz E, Van Doren M. TPAPN offers extraordinary volunteer opportunity. Texas Board of Nursing Bulletin 2011;42(2):5.

ADVOCACY FOR NURSES: PROGRAMMATIC

The desire to participate as an advocate is only the first step. There is an application and committee review process, a training program, and a continuing education requirement. Approval of advocates is made jointly by the case management staff and the Advocate Committee. In addition to emotional support, advocates provide guidance through the TPAPN process, which includes a myriad of forms, scheduled interviews, and a structured protocol that includes drug testing associated with returning to work. The most successful participants are those who are enthusiastic about their recovery and are committed to following the process responsibly. The support of advocates is a significant factor in the participant's success.

The success of a nursing peer assistance program has much to do with its own organizational structure, policies, and internal programs. Support from the state legislature and the Board of Nursing is essential. In addition, there must be enthusiasm for the program among nursing professionals; participants and advocates who believe in its value and potential for success.[6]

Nurses who are interested in becoming advocates must submit an application that includes their promise to uphold TPAPN's advocate standards of practice, disclose their personal experience with SUD or psychiatric disorder, and address their beliefs regarding the treatment of SUDs and psychiatric disorders among nurses. Applicants must acknowledge that they have the time and energy needed for active participation. The application includes a letter of reference from a professional colleague and a summary of their work history. Applications are reviewed by the case management staff and the Advocate Committee comprising regional and at-large advocates. Final approval is predicated on attending the TPAPN advocate training. There are ongoing educational requirements beyond the required in-house training; advocates must attend a certified educational activity pertaining to some aspect of SUD or psychiatric disorder every 3 years.

The Advocate Committee is composed of 8 regional and at-large members appointed from the active advocacy pool. Besides approving applicants for advocacy, the Advocate Committee also assists with the annual strategic planning and certain aspects of program development pertinent to advocates. This group also serves as a peer review committee under the Texas Nurse Practice Act, should concerns or complaints be received about TPAPN nurse volunteers while discharging their duties as advocates. One member of the Advocacy Committee also serves on the program's Advisory Committee composed of representatives of statewide nursing organizations and specialty practice groups, which gives input to the Board of Directors related to budget, strategic planning, and organizational development.

Peer assistance organizations promote patient safety, assist nurses in need, promote professional competency and accountability, and enhance the just culture in our health care workplaces. Mary Grayson (2012) aptly reflects this need: "…if we take care of our employees, all else will follow…and that includes their mental health".[7]

REFERENCES

1. Simko S. A doctor's ordinary labor can provide extraordinary mercy. In Texas Children's Blog. 2012. Available at: http://www.texaschildrensblog.org/2012/03/a-doctors-ordinary-labor-can-provide-extraordinary-mercy/. Accessed September 28, 2012.
2. ANA Code of Ethics (American Nurses Association, 2001).
3. The profession's response to the problem of addictions and psychiatric disorders in nursing (American Nurses Association, 2002).

4. National Council of State Boards of Nursing. Substance use disorder in nursing: a resource manual and guidelines for alternative and disciplinary monitoring programs. Chicago: National Council of State Boards of Nursing; 2011.
5. Bartholomew K. End nurse-to-nurse hostility: why nurses eat their young and each other. Marblehead (MA): HCPro; 2006.
6. Tipton PH. Predictors of relapse for nurses participating in a peer assistance program. Denton, Texas: Unpublished doctoral dissertation, Texas Women's University; 2005.
7. Grayson M. Taking care of our own. Hospital and Health Network, 2012. Available at: http://www.hhnmag.com/hhnmag_app/jsp/articledisplay.jsp?dcrpath=HHNMAG/Article/data/05MAY2012/0512HHN_ednotes&domain=HHNMAG. Accessed June 1, 2012.

Advocacy for the Older Patient

Mary Nouvertne Klein, RN, MSN, LNFA

KEYWORDS

• Older persons • Gerontology • Aging • Nurses • Care

KEY POINTS

- Nurses advocating for older patients can help them deal effectively with the maze of insensitive territory, endless questions, and unexplained testing.
- As the number of elderly patients increases, there is a greater need for experience in gerontology in all medical and nursing specialties.
- Good preoperative planning includes an effective transition of care from the hospital to home, reducing the potential for complications and rehospitalization.
- Older adults are particularly sensitive to medications, which must be aggressively reviewed so that unnecessary drugs are eliminated and dosages are adjusted for optimal effect.

INTRODUCTION

Older persons with health issues succumb to an obscure maze of insensitive territory, revealing personal information to strangers who are looking at a computer screen, and enduring seemingly endless unexplained testing. Older patients trust the doctor who has ordered the tests, treatment, and/or hospitalization. However, losing track of what has already been done and what yet needs to be done is common. Navigating the ever-changing health care system can be a challenge even for a healthy, independent, younger adult. For the older patient, the system can be very confusing, intimidating, and frustrating, and the lack of control can result in adverse outcomes (**Box 1**).

"Baby boomers," born in the years following World War II, are now turning 65 years of age. This large, independent group of people with a great deal of social influence has changed the perception of the older population. Getting older is considered more as a time of independence, activity, and productivity; fewer people believe that aging leads to a helpless, childlike, and unproductive time of life. Preventive health efforts and medical advancements contribute to living healthier and much longer lives. Societal pressure to look younger has led to a tremendous market for anti-aging remedies; people spend a lot of money on plastic surgery, cosmetics, and nutritional supplements. The physical and cosmetic changes that occur with aging are too often portrayed as an illness rather than a natural progression of life. Looking younger does not prevent the

Retired
E-mail address: mkleinhome@sbcglobal.net

Perioperative Nursing Clinics 7 (2012) 447–459
http://dx.doi.org/10.1016/j.cpen.2012.08.010

Box 1
Causes of fragmentation and changes in care delivery for older patient

1. The number of patients older than 65 years is increasing steadily, and health care needs increase with age, yet there is less provider reimbursement. Lengthy office visits are impractical, leaving patients with less information and fewer resources for navigating the health care system effectively. Some doctors are opting-out entirely of seeing older patients who have limited insurance.

2. New regulations require the primary physician to perform standard screening and preventive education during office visits, which is confusing for patients who come to the office expecting only treatment.

3. Primary physicians often refer to specialists. A patient with multiple diagnoses may be seeing many different physicians at the same time, making it difficult to coordinate effective and efficient care.

4. Electronic medical records (EMR) are often not compatible with the software used by the patient's variety of physicians. Mistakes that occur when inputting information may not be corrected.

5. There is often poor coordination of care. For example, when a patient is admitted to a hospital via the emergency room, a physician hospitalist who is managing the patient for the first time may order repeat tests, change or add treatments and medications, or inadvertently refer the patient to new physicians for follow-up after discharge.

6. Information can be lost or misinterpreted as it is passed between physician and patient, patient and family, family and physician, and physician to physician. Treatments can be overlooked; medications can be mismanaged. The side effects of excessive or missing medications and drug interactions account for many visits to the emergency department and hospital admissions.

7. Hearing loss, impaired vision, memory problems, and other disabilities can complicate care and interfere with clear communication. Simple problems can escalate rapidly, jeopardizing the patient's overall health.

8. Government insurers are exploring measures to consolidate and reduce costs associated with caring for the elderly.

---

physiologic aging of our internal organs, brain, nervous system, and skeletal structure; however, proper nutrition, exercise, avoiding addictive behaviors, and advancing medical technology have slowed aging significantly. Chronic illnesses, such as diabetes, lung disease, heart disease, cancer, and bone degeneration, that were once debilitating and deadly can now be successfully treated and sometimes cured.

The health care arena is attempting to address the advancing median age of the patient population. Many medical and nursing school curricula include some geriatric education; yet the number of physicians and advanced practice nurses specializing in geriatric care is not increasing. Despite the dedicated practitioners and improvements in treatment protocols, there is an obvious need for improvement in the way the geriatric patient is managed.

Jo is a 71 year-old active, very intelligent grandmother who raised a family as a single working mother. She is a licensed boat captain who charters overnight trips and teaches sailing. In her 50s, she earned her private airplane pilot's license. She exercises regularly and religiously schedules her well-health checks. She also cares for an aging mother and a daughter-in-law who has cancer. In the last few years, Jo developed chronic back issues and was referred to an orthopedist, neurologist, and pain specialist who ordered several conflicting treatments. Although she can navigate a boat and a plane through sets of complex

procedures, she describes navigating health care between physicians and treat-
ments confusing and sometimes overwhelming. She does not hesitate to call
a close friend who is a Registered Nurse for advice and support.

Many of the elderly can remember when the family doctor treated every illness the patient and his family had from "cradle to grave"; when the entire family enjoyed a long-term relationship with their physician. Care was continued from the office to the hospital and even to the operating room. Decisions about treatment were collaborative and involved psychosocial, personal, ethical, and financial issues. Many doctors would like to be loyal patient advocates, but the current health care system makes that type of practice financially difficult to attain.

The health care system is becoming more fragmented, less convenient, and less responsive to the needs of older patients. The quality of the long-term relationship between physician and patient has eroded. Visits are hurried and less personal. More medical treatment decisions are now being made by the specialist physician rather than the primary doctor. Patients are expected to take more control of scheduling appointments, tracking test results, and organizing care needs. In reality, health care at present, particularly for elderly patients, feels much less caring and friendly, and lacks cohesiveness and coordination. Many nurses are aware of this and are trying to help the older patient population.

The nursing profession continues to provide compassionate care and has a much greater opportunity to develop relationships with patients. Nurses specializing in geriatric patient care have recognized the need for cohesiveness and continuity. Nurses have developed new assessment tools, nursing guidelines, and advocacy programs for the aging patient population. Any nurse, regardless of their area of practice, can help advocate for change to improve access to and quality of care for older patients.

THE OLDER SURGICAL PATIENT

More than one-half of all operations in the United States are performed on older patients. Medicare is the primary health insurance for most Americans older than 65 years and for younger people with disabilities. Medicare is administered by the federal government and funded by taxes on income and premium payments from recipients. The number of recipients on Medicare is increasing, and the medical costs are also continually increasing. Measures to reduce health care costs include requiring more surgical procedures to be performed in ambulatory facilities that are overall less expensive to perform than hospital procedures. As a result, ambulatory centers are increasing in number and the hospital outpatient surgery departments are expanding.

In recent years, great efforts have been made to improve outpatient care. With shorter-acting and more effective anesthetic agents and advancements in minimally invasive surgical techniques and instrumentation, many successful operations and life-saving procedures are now safely performed on people who are in their 80s and 90s. Avoiding hospital stays can actually prevent costly complications, such as urinary tract infections, isolation delirium, pressure sores, and falls.

An outpatient surgical procedure for an older person can involve time to get second opinions, clearance from several different physicians, and time to schedule preoperative testing. Arrangements might be necessary for help at home postoperatively by rearranging furniture, organizing transportation, and obtaining medical equipment needed in the home. The challenges are especially difficult for the older patients who are reluctant to ask for help, and for those whose family members live at a distance, or who cannot be available for an extended period of time.

Outpatient procedures are most often scheduled by the operating physician's office, which the patient may have visited only once, and with which the patient has no established relationship. There is usually a call from the hospital or outpatient facility several days before an elective procedure to tell the patient what medications to take or not take, how long before surgery to stop eating and drinking, to be sure that someone is available to take them home after surgery and that someone will remain with them for the first 12 to 24 h after receiving anesthesia.

The first real nursing assessment and focused teaching the patient receives may be just before the procedure. Not only is this process often an insufficient preparation for an elderly patient but also standard assessment tools are frequently inadequate for the older population. A geriatric assessment is designed to collect information on the medical, psychosocial, and functional capabilities and limitations of an older patient. Geriatric assessment differs from a standard assessment in that it focuses on the elderly with multiple diagnoses, emphasizes functional status and quality of life, and determines if other disciplines (social worker, home health, and physical therapy) need to be involved for a successful treatment outcome.

Diagnosis alone does not determine a patient's quality of life or the outcome of a surgery. A patient from a nursing home may have the same diagnosis as a seemingly healthy working older adult. All too frequently, however, an older patient, discharged after an outpatient procedure, is admitted several days later because of a fall, medication mix-up, or inadequate home care. Even though, the incidence of surgical complications is greater in the older patient, secondary complications may be even more devastating and costly. The efficiency of ambulatory surgery may not provide adequate time to assess, communicate with, and prepare older patients.

Mrs E.N. lived independently in a senior housing village and at 90 years was scheduled for routine cataract surgery as an outpatient. She had stiff joints and untreated severe hearing loss but was otherwise alert and healthy. When she was asked before surgery if she had help, she said "yes, my neighbor is going to assist me." The 85-year-old female neighbor drove her to the center, waited, and dropped her off at home after the operation. Within a few hours, Mrs E.N. got lightheaded, fell, and was unable to reach the phone for help. Her neighbor found her later in the day and called an ambulance. The emergency department ruled out serious injury, and she was sent home. She was unable to properly direct the eye drops and possibly due to confusion or from the fall, she never regained vision in that eye.

Mrs H., aged 69 years, underwent outpatient surgery for the replacement of a kidney dialysis port in her arm. While being transferred from a stretcher to a bed she sustained a large skin tear on her leg. The injury was not noticed by the staff and the patient did not think it was important enough to bother someone. Several days after discharge, the skin tear became infected, and she required a hospital admission and extended stay for intravenous antibiotics.

Mrs B, an active, alert 90-year-old pianist, had an outpatient partial second-toe amputation for circulatory issues. She received a local anesthesia. Her 86-year-old husband had driven her to the hospital outpatient department for the simple procedure, and she was discharged home on pain medication. Within a few days, she became very constipated and her husband began giving her water enemas. Because the toe was painful, she continued to take the pain medication along with her other medications she had been receiving for past-treated ovarian cancer. Mrs B. soon become very confused would not eat or get out of bed and talked about dying. Her husband called their daughter-in-law, a retired nurse, who contacted the primary doctor. The doctor ordered lab work and discovered her sodium level was very low. He called her oncologist and she was admitted to the cancer hospital for testing and intravenous fluids. She was discharged home after 48 hours but readmitted to the general hospital by her practitioner for fever two days later. Still confused, she received a computed tomographic scan ordered by a neurologist and reacted to the dye. After ten days, still confused and not walking, she was discharged to a skilled nursing unit for restorative care. There, a geriatrician found out about the water enemas that probably caused her electrolyte imbalance and properly treated her constipation. He also reduced her medications. After two months of skilled care, she improved significantly and was discharged home alert and walking. She went back to playing the piano at a senior center. The toe healed and her ovarian cancer remained in remission until her peaceful death three years later.

OLDER PATIENTS HAVE MORE COMPLEX HEALTH ISSUES

Medication-related problems are common, yet preventable. Many hospital admissions are related to the effects of anticoagulants and diabetic, heart, and pain medications. Often medications are prescribed for the side effects of other medications. Pain medication for the elderly postoperative patients must be managed with care. Many older patients with chronic conditions take multiple prescription medications. Confusion in managing medications is not uncommon. Determining the cognitive status of any patient before and after surgery can avoid a major setback in recovery. Delirium or temporary reversible confusion can be caused by medications, anesthesia, infection, dehydration, or electrolyte imbalance. Undiagnosed delirium can lead to imbalance, falls, and fractures.

Mrs D, an alert 79-year-old independent woman with some memory loss underwent a partial mastectomy as an outpatient for removal of a breast mass. Except for pain management and dressing changes, no further treatment was planned. She was to continue on her routine medications for hypertension, high cholesterol, and type II diabetes. Prior to discharge the daughter was concerned about her postoperative confusion and was told by the nurse it was probably from the anesthesia and she should improve. She was cleared to go home. Once home, the confusion worsened. Mrs D. was unable to properly care for herself or communicate effectively with her elderly husband who also had some memory issues. The confusion was addressed with the surgeon at the postoperative visit and he referred her to a neurologist who diagnosed Alzheimer disease. The daughter admitted her to an assisted living facility for safety and she passed away within ten months.

THE PERIOPERATIVE NURSE ADVOCATE

Nurses are natural advocates for older patients. Nurses often take the initiative to promote and provide better care for older patients. Many factors place patients, including the elderly, at risk for less than optimal care. No monetary incentive for hospitals and doctors to reduce the number of unnecessary surgeries, or to prevent admissions is available. Older patients are frequently directed to the emergency department for minor issues because the doctor's office is busy, or it is after-hours and the patient does not know what else to do. Nurse advocates for older patients are working toward better continuity of care, more comprehensive geriatric assessments, and reform measures to keep older patients away from redundant testing, unneeded procedures, and avoidable hospital admissions.

Our society focuses on healthy aging. One of the hardest things for an older person to do is admit to needing help, and one of the biggest fears is losing their independence. A move to a nursing facility is often viewed as a punishment or a place to die. Often an elderly spouse caring for a wife or husband with a disability, dementia, or Alzheimer disease will ignore the need for assistance. An older caregiver may not want to burden family members or to risk being placed in a nursing facility. Caregivers delay their own treatment when they become ill or need surgery. Stress is associated with caring for a needy spouse; sometimes the relationship becomes abusive. When working with the elderly, discussing their home life, assessing for the sources of anxiety, and looking for signs of abuse or neglect is necessary.

Living alone after the death of a spouse can be very difficult for the elderly. Family members may or may not be sensitive to their needs. There may be no family close by or no family at all. Denial intensifies with fear of losing independence. The patient may not tell the physician or any of their family members all the issues and depression and/or self-neglect may be missed.

Mrs N., aged 73 years lived alone for two years after her husband died suddenly. Her son and daughter lived in other states. While visiting, the daughter noticed her mother's excessive mail-order buying, inability to balance her checkbook, cook or clean house, and confusion with her many medications. The mother assured her everything was fine. She was being treated for hypertension, seizure disorder, and high cholesterol, and she had a pacemaker for heart block. Concerned about medication overdose or dementia, the daughter scheduled an appointment with her neurologist. The neurologist performed a mini-mental examination, which the mother passed. He casually informed the daughter there was no problem and her medications were necessary. He refused to speak to the daughter privately because he said it violated patient-doctor confidentiality, even though the daughter was a Registered Nurse. The next few years involved numerous hospital admissions for seizures, increased medication dosages, and the addition of new medications. Neighbors became concerned and the daughter decided to move her mother to senior housing near her. Mrs N.'s seizures continued and she was not taking care of herself.

After a long hospitalization during which medications were added to her regimen, Ms N was diagnosed with a new seizure disorder and moderate-to-severe dementia. She stopped walking and was unable to feed herself. It was recommended that she be placed in a nursing home. After a thorough assessment, the professional staff at the nursing home reevaluated her medications, eliminating some and reducing the dosages of others. Her improvement was so dramatic that she was able to provide most of her own care and was relocated to an assisted living facility. For the next nine years she walked everywhere and was self-sufficient. She had successful outpatient cataract surgeries and a pacemaker change. She chose to stay in assisted living because she liked the people, calling them "her new family". Although she is now in a wheelchair and has significant memory loss, she remains aware of her surroundings.

The elderly are faced with many decisions involving living arrangements, transportation, medical treatments, and financial issues. Sometimes, preventive measures are delayed or refused and a sudden health crisis or accident creates an abrupt change. When the elderly cannot make effective decisions, intervention is necessary. The quantity and character of intervention depends individual needs, and very few situations are alike. Often the elderly individual is more focused on losing independence than on the situation itself, and interventions by others are perceived as undesirable.

There is a tremendous need for nurses educated in caring for older patients, particularly in the outpatient surgical setting, in which a comprehensive assessment is critical to determining the appropriate care for each patient. Nurses often sense that an older patient's needs may be greater than the issue on which the physician is

---

The author's story

I was destined to be a geriatric nurse. When I was young I was sent to take care of my grand-mother who died a painful death from breast cancer. I also lived next door to a nursing home and worked in the kitchen after school and on weekends during high school. Some of the residents often helped me clean up and I got to know them very well. We were like family and I enjoyed their company.

After high school, I became a nursing assistant, and a supervisor encouraged me to go to nursing school. I graduated from a Diploma School of Nursing, then earned my bachelor of science in nursing. To my surprise, I was the only student who signed up for the geriatric elective. I earned my master of science in nursing in a new geriatric nursing program at the University of Texas School of Nursing. After a number of years of intensive care nursing, and office-based nursing while in school, I accepted a position managing my first hospital-based geriatric skilled Medi-care unit. I became well known throughout the hospital as the geriatric advisor and advocate. I assisted in developing new policies and procedures for older acute care patients, and advo-cated for rehabilitative and restorative care for the geriatric skilled-care patients. My next posi-tion was hospital-based transitional care regional consultant, and I had the privilege of starting up new skilled Medicare units in Texas, Mississippi, and Virginia.

A miracle pregnancy forced me to be a stay-at-home mother for my newborn twins. I welcomed my new position. Like many mothers, I became involved in local community, church, and school activities and found myself more involved with older people than I could have imagined. Caring for my mother-in-law introduced me to the difficulties older patients faced outside of acute care and nursing facilities. I became a resident consultant for extended family, friends, and acquaintances who approached me to discuss issues with their aging parents, issues involving medications, falls, confusion, Alzheimer disease, finding caregivers, disappointment with doctors, complications from operations, confusion over the many different levels of long-term care, and end-of-life care.

I discovered gaps in our medical care system between diagnosis, treatment, discharge, and rehabilitation. On many occasions, I was disappointed with my mother's treatment in the emer-gency department and hospital. My mother-in-law's pain medications caused her to go into respiratory failure. My grandmother's complications after outpatient surgery made me realize that, no matter how good the hospital care might be, without appropriate follow-up care at home, disastrous complications can result. My personal experiences have made me an enthusi-astic advocate for appropriate care for the elderly.

Like many of my colleagues, I am caring for an aging parent. It is a daunting challenge to find care or an appropriate living situation for an aging parent who needs attention. I firmly believe nurses are the foundation for successful care and treatment of older patients. Maintaining connections with my nurse friends and meeting with other advocates for the aging population is invigorating. As Agatha Christie says "I like living. I have sometimes been wildly, despairingly, acutely miserable, racked with sorrow, but through it all, I still know quite certainly that just to be alive is a grand thing."

---

focused. Perioperative nurses have the unique ability to develop a trusting relationship with patients and gather a wealth of pertinent information in short time. Nurses can apprise the physician of issues that affect the patients' ability to care for themselves. They may recommend rescheduling a surgery or advise when an older patient should spend the night in the hospital. Nurses usually expedite the order for home health, social services, or physical therapy. Perioperative nurses are in the best position to perform a great service to a vulnerable population.

HOW TO BE AN ADVOCATE FOR YOUR OLDER PATIENTS
Be Proactive in Improving the Delivery of Care to the Older Patients in Your Care
There are some excellent resources available to help perioperative nurses get started (**Boxes 2** and **3**). The Nurses Improving Care for Healthsystem Elders (NICHE)

Box 2
Resources for nurses caring for older adult patients

The Hartford Institute for Geriatric Nursing

www.hartfordign.org 212-992-9416

Began in 1996 to improve the quality of care of older adults through excellence in nursing practice, research, education, and advocacy policy. The Hartford Institute for Geriatric Nursing provides access to the following programs:

Nurses Improving Care for Healthsystem elders

www.nicheprogram.org

Focus is on improving staff competence in caring for older patients and supporting the implementation of hospital geriatric protocols. Provides extensive resources and tools that guide, support, and educate health care professionals and facilities. Goal is to improve patient, family, and staff satisfaction rates by providing quality care. At present, has more than 300 hospital members.

ConsultGeriRN

www.consultgerirn.org

Provides nurses and other health care professionals immediate access to geriatric care information. Comprehensive geriatric assessments and tools are provided. Information is kept current and obtained from evidence-based research and practice. Continuing education contact hours available.

eLearing Center

www.hartfordign.org

A continuing education site for courses, tools, and other resources with the objective of improving care of older adults in clinical settings. Also provides the resources for nurses interested in taking the gerontological certification examination.

Coalition of Geriatric Nursing Organizations

www.hartfordign.org/advocacy/cgno/

Began in 2001. Represents approximately 29,000 nurses from nursing specialty organizations that provide geriatric care in a variety of settings. Goal is to promote a health care environment for older adults that reflect accessibility, evidence-based practice and high quality person-centered care.

The American Geriatric Society

www.americangeritrics.org

A not-for-profit organization of health professionals interested in the health, independence, and quality of life of older people. This organization provides leadership and advocacy to healthcare professionals, policy makers, and the public.

National Association of Geriatric Nurses

www.ngna.org

Dedicated to improving the clinical care of older adults. Membership involves all levels of nursing in various practice settings.

---

www.nicheprogram.org.is an advocacy program developed by the Hartford Institute of Geriatric Nursing to enhance hospital care for all patients older than 65 years. Encourage your facility to join NICHE. The organization focuses on assuring quality care with successful outcomes in all levels of patient care. NICHE nurses have developed the Rights of the Older Hospitalized Patient. Evidence-based best practice

---

Box 3
Advocacy resources for patients and families

The Alzheimer's Association www.alz.org

American Association of Retired Persons www.aarp.org

The National Center on Elder Abuse www.ncea.aoa.gov

Kaiser Health News www.kaiserhealthnews.org

National Citizens Coalition for Nursing Home Reform www.nccnhr.org

National Area Agency on Aging www.n4a.org

National Institute on Aging www.nia.nih.org

National Council on Aging www.ncoa.org

Nursing Home Compare www.Medicare.gov

Nurses Improving Care for Healthsystem Elders www.nichprogram.org

---

models are available for institutions to use in developing their own programs for improving care to older patients, including a complete guide to the comprehensive geriatric assessment. The site contains a multitude of resources for nurses and managers Encourage your facility or department to hire a nurse with a specialty in gerontology to educate staff members, assist in assessing older patients, and coordinate follow-up care at home. A preoperative and postoperative home assessment can identify potential problems and promote more effective patient management.

The American Geriatrics Society (www.americangeriatric.org) has developed The Beers Criteria for Potentially Inappropriate Medication Use in Older Adults, that identifies medications requiring reduced dosages or that should be avoided in older patients. This list should be readily available at your facility.

Expand Your Knowledge

Avail yourself of educational opportunities focused on care of the elderly. The Association of Perioperative Nurses (AORN) www.aorn.org offers a wealth of clinical resources and continuing education targeting caring for older adults in the perioperative setting. The National Gerontological Nursing Association (http://www.ngna.org/) is a comprehensive Web site for nurses needing information about managing elderly patients. Many other specialty nursing organizations have resources for managing the care of older patients in their specialty.

The Hartford Institute for Geriatric Nursing's Web site, ConsultGeriRN (www.ConsultGeriRN.com), is an excellent instant resource. The site houses clinical tools, continuing education, specialty-specific geriatric resources, and advocacy information. The site includes webinars, assessment tools, and demonstration. The *Try This* series features a two-page document with a description of why each topic is important when caring for older patients on the first page, and an assessment tool that can be administered in 20 minutes or less on the second page. *Try This* instruments are designed to be screening tools and not for diagnosis. The *Try This* series also includes the Fulmer SPICES overall assessment tool for older adults.

Expand your learning beyond your immediate setting. Take a tour of a hospital rehabilitation and skilled unit. Find a geriatric nurse you can call when you have questions about an elderly patient. Get to know the social workers associated with your facility. Social workers help with resources for patients who need home health, caregivers, assisted living, nursing home, and support group information. Although the social worker addresses many inpatients, they are less apt to be called for an outpatient. This may even require a change in the hospital policy.

Visit an elderly person in a nursing facility. Volunteer at a senior center. Once you have a better understanding of how the older population lives, you will develop a more comprehensive view and greater satisfaction in caring for them. Your elderly patients can teach you many things from their own experiences. The relationship you develop with your older patients will not only be meaningful and educational but will also provide valuable information that will facilitate a successful surgical outcome.

Be Aware of the Public Policy Issues Related to the Elderly
Follow the legislative activity targeting health care for older patients. Both state and federal legislatures continue to debate the cost of health care for the aging population and its effect on the state and the nation. Being a member of nursing and nursing specialty professional organizations can keep you informed about the impact of legislative activity on patients and on the profession. Nursing organizations' Web sites usually provide the step-by-step process for contacting your legislatures and lobbying for changes. The American Association for Retired Persons and National Council on Aging are public advocacy organizations that lobby for better elder care.

Learn How to Overcome Barriers and Communicate with an Older Patient
Speaking directly to the patient helps you gain trust and also helps to assess their ability to understand. Be aware of limitations; for instance, when the patient has vision or hearing impairment, gently touch the patient's hand to let them know you are there. Allow the older patient to speak and finish what they are trying to say. Speaking to the patient in lower tones and more slowly helps them understand you. Shouting is offensive and not all elderly patients are hearing impaired.

Focus on the patient, not just the surgical procedure. Always explain what you are going to do. Family members occasionally take too much control and do not allow the patient to speak or make or participate in decision-making. A family member doing all the talking should be asked to wait until you are finished speaking with the patient. Make sure that the patient understands a document such as the Informed Consent before they sign it.

If a patient is not completely competent, be sure that they have a legal guardian. When the patient seems confused, speak to the family member/companion away from the patient to gather more information. Do not object to a family member wanting to speak with you alone; this is not a violation of the Health Insurance Portability and Accountability Act if it helps to gather relevant patient assessment information. Use your best judgment. Caregivers should not hesitate to use appropriate touch to connect with the older patient. Also remember that, even though a patient appears confused or has received sedation, he or she may still be very aware of what you are saying.

Mrs R was an 82-year-old independent lady who avoided doctors. She was a former smoker who underwent an outpatient bronchoscopy and lung biopsy at a major medical center hospital. She was very nervous but was assured that this was a quick procedure and she would be released shortly. However, once Mrs R. was in the operating room, the computer malfunctioned. Without giving the patient an explanation, the technicians and nurses were in and out of the room talking frantically, and the surgeon left to see another patient, while waiting for the repair. It was more than an hour and a half before a new machine was brought in. The procedure went well and Mrs R. was taken to the recovery room extremely upset, stating that no one knew what they were doing and the doctors and nurses kept leaving her alone in the room. She feared that something had gone wrong with her procedure and no one was telling her. The recovery nurse was unaware of the computer failure, and assumed she was confused from the anesthesia. Only when the family questioned the doctor did they find out about the computer failure that had occurred in the operating room. The hospital's patient representative also researched the situation and found that Mrs R's description was accurate. Once Mrs R was apprised of the situation, she became much calmer, but was still angry. She stated, "I will never come here again." The lung biopsy was negative but to this day she recalls the horrible event and has chosen other facilities and physicians for her health care.

Speak Up

Speaking up can be difficult for the nurse when the patient is scheduled to be in the operating room, and the nurse's recommendation disrupts the schedule. However, the nurse may be the first one to assess an issue that can have a major impact on the patient's well-being. Be an advocate and speak up for your patient. Issues are better resolved before surgery than to risk complications that could have been avoided. Older patients should be treated as if they were your own parents.

If your patient mentions a problem at home, has had recent falls, or seems confused or upset, further assessment is needed. Further assessment is also needed if the patient or person with them does not seem to understand the directions for postoperative care. If the patient appears unprepared or you believe that the situation seems overwhelming to the patient, speak up. Delaying or canceling a procedure may prevent an adverse outcome created by the lack of resources or continuity of care.

Teach Your Older Adult Patients, Your Parents, Family Members, and Friends to Be Proactive and Responsible for Their Own Care with These Tips

Take charge of your own health care: Have your own file

Patients cannot rely on doctors and hospitals to keep track of all their test results, doctors, medications, and needs. Keeping your own file with all diagnoses, medications, surgeries, current laboratory and test results reduces communication errors. For the tech-savvy, there are programs available to help patients maintain their own health history, medication records, and doctor appointments. Ideally, these programs download and upload test results instantly if they are compatible with doctor's offices. Keep advanced directives, important legal documents, and any special information handy. During an emergency this information could save the patient's life.

Write down all questions before a doctor's visit

Many patients have some level of anxiety when visiting a doctor. Doctor's have limited time, but usually take time to answer all questions the patient asks during the visit. Don't hesitate to share with the physician your list of concerns. It is more effective to give and receive all the necessary information while you have a doctor's full attention; calling the office later with a forgotten question does not always produce satisfactory results.

Always bring paper and pen or an electronic pad to all doctor's visits. Capture the answers to the questions asked and all of the pertinent information given. Information can be missed or forgotten, especially if you are not feeling well and it's hard to concentrate. Small mishaps can turn into big issues. If new medications are prescribed, make sure you determine if previous medications need to be discontinued and if the new medications are compatible with the ones currently being taken. Ideally, the person accompanying the elderly patient takes notes while the patient gives the physician his undivided attention.

Take advantage of the online information available
Learn about your illness before your doctor visit. Massive amount of information is available on the Internet about every disease and many types of treatments. Talk to others you know with the same illness. Know the options that are available for treatment. Ask for nondrug interventions, which encourages a healthier discussion with your doctor and allow the opportunity to discusst the best treatment option for you and why some may or may not work. This discussion also rules out deceptive information you have come across on the Internet.

Bring all your prescription and nonprescription medications, vitamins, herbal remedies, and so forth to all initial doctors' visits
Although many patients have heard this over and over, few older patients actually bring all their medications to the doctor. Balance problems, dizziness, hearing loss, incontinence, dehydration, falls, fractures, and car accidents have all been traced back to the improper use of medications. Always ask if there are medications you can stop taking. Inform the doctor if they are too expensive. Multiple drug prescriptions from various doctors are a huge problem and the cause of many visits to the emergency department and admissions to the hospital. Never assume the doctors have communicated with each other.

If you are taking narcotic medications for chronic pain, it is best to ask a spouse, family member or companion to be a part of your treatment. Together, keep track of your pain level and how much pain medication you are taking. Be honest with your doctor about the side-effects you are having. Larger doses may not be tolerated as you get older and different strategies should be tried to control your pain. In combination with antidepressants and antianxiety medications, narcotic dosages should be adjusted. Alcohol use interferes with medications. Be sure to be honest with your doctor about how much alcohol you drink daily.

When referred to a specialist, provide a complete picture of your health status
Do not count on the referring physician to provide all the information to the specialist. Their communication may have been a short phone call weeks before your appointment.

Prepare adequately for a surgical procedure
Arrange for someone to stay with you for as long as necessary. Make arrangements for someone to run errands, take care of your spouse, cook meals, and clean. Arrange for a competent, trusted relative or friend to accompany you to your preoperative and postoperative assessments as well as on the day of surgery. If a hospital admission is necessary, have someone stay with you. Most hospitals accommodate someone in your room. Hospital staff is not always readily available to help you to the bathroom, or with other immediate needs. Having someone keep track of information from the nurses and doctors and therapists is very helpful. Too often their visits go unknown to you because you are drowsy or sleeping. Always keep in the back of your mind that hospitals can be dangerous places for infections, falling, overmedicating, and errors. To have someone with you at all times for your safety is the best option. Friends and family can take shifts if you have an extended stay. The better the communication, the better the care and the quicker the discharge.

SUMMARY

Good preoperative planning includes an effective transition of care from the hospital to home, reducing the potential for complications and rehospitalization. Medications must be aggressively reviewed, unnecessary drugs eliminated, and dosages adjusted for optimal effect. Communication between practitioners and treatment centers needs to improve.

Most perioperative nurses care for a large number of older patients but do not have specific training in assessing the geriatric patients. Assessing an older patient requires more time and requires a different approach from younger adults. Using specialized, comprehensive geriatric assessment tools is more efficient to identify areas of concern unique to the older adult. A focused assessment can help older patients avoid dangerous complications after surgery.

The percentage of elderly people in our population is increasing. Our society values healthy aging and preventing the disabilities associated with getting older. There will be an increasing demand for improved services and advancements in treatment protocols. Health care reform is focusing on reducing costs and increasing access, but the elderly present a challenge. There are not enough doctors and nurses specializing in the care of the elderly. Gerontology must be incorporated early into all medical and nursing programs. At present, geriatric nurses are taking an active role in helping older patients through the development of advocacy organizations, evidence-based research, and providing continuing education opportunities for all nurses in caring for the older patient.

Advocating for the Pediatric Patient

Aracely Lucendo Díaz, DUE[a,b,*]

KEYWORDS

- Advocacy • Pediatric patient care • Patient rights

KEY POINTS

- Pediatric surgical patients represent a small percentage of the surgical patient population, and perioperative nurses try to be sensitive to their unique needs.
- Pediatric surgery spans a variety of specialties.
- Nurses often face challenges caring for pediatric surgical patients within a tertiary hospital, but try to address those obstacles as creatively as possible.

INTRODUCTION

The author works in the Hospital Universitario de Canarias (HUC), a public, tertiary care, 761-bed university hospital in Tenerife, Canary Islands, Spain. The hospital serves a population of nearly 500,000 and is a referral hospital for the Canary Islands for all specialties. It is the only referral center for renopancreatic transplants from living donors, and has recently been designated a reference center of the National Health Service for pancreas transplants.

Although the hospital has dedicated resources for children including a pediatric admission area, a pediatric unit, a pediatric outpatient unit with 17 rooms with a waiting room specifically designed for children, four treatment rooms, and a pediatric intensive care unit with specialized care for premature infants, there is no dedicated area for children in the surgical suite.

Pediatric surgical patients represent a small percentage of the surgical patient population, and the perioperative nurses try to be sensitive to the unique needs of pediatric patients while working within hospital protocols. Children and adults share the same preanesthesia area, attire, and recovery area. Pediatric surgery spans a variety of specialties and there are no dedicated pediatric operating rooms. This arrangement scatters the resources for pediatric patients throughout the surgical suite and makes preparing for a pediatric case somewhat of a challenge. There are also no perioperative

[a] Hospital Universitario de Canarias, Ctra. Ofra S/N La Cuesta, 38320 La Laguna, Tenerife, Canary Islands, Spain; [b] Nursing College of Santa Cruz de Tenerife, Tenerife, Canary Islands, Spain
* Corresponding author. Hospital Universitario de Canarias, Ctra. Ofra S/N La Cuesta, 38320 La Laguna, Tenerife, Canary Islands, Spain
E-mail address: aracelylucendodiaz@gmail.com

Perioperative Nursing Clinics 7 (2012) 461–469
http://dx.doi.org/10.1016/j.cpen.2012.08.001   periopnursing.theclinics.com
1556-7931/12/$ – see front matter © 2012 Elsevier Inc. All rights reserved.

nurses dedicated to the care of pediatric patients. The nurses at HUC address these obstacles as creatively as they can.

Preparation for this article included an extensive literature search including the United Nations "Convention on the Rights of the Child," (CRC) which provides a comprehensive framework of rights that facilitates a holistic approach to promote the well-being of children. Documents from the World Health Organization, UNICEF, and the European Union also speak to the specialized care to which patients under 19 are entitled. This article presents the author's recommendations to perioperative managers and caregivers for overcoming the barriers to sensitive and appropriate care of pediatric patients in an adult environment.

WHAT BARRIERS DO WE FACE?
Surgical suite design
HUC lacks a suitable area to welcome children to the operating room. This increases anxiety for children and parents. Children coming to surgery from the pediatric unit leave an area with bright-colored walls, nurses in cheerful uniforms, familiar toys, familiar faces, and the privilege of having their parents at the bedside. Before entering the surgical suite, they are taken from their parents to a room that is cold and clinical with unfamiliar smells, the atmosphere is efficient and serious, and there are adult patients in varying degrees of distress. Everything is strange and frightening. Even if the parents are able to accompany the child to the preanesthesia area, their reaction to the environment is as uncomfortable as their children's.

Psychological preparation for children and parents
Numerous studies speak of the importance of preparation of parents and children for a surgical procedure. Healthcare facilities are encouraged to develop tools to address the specific needs of the pediatric population. In reality, many pediatric patients and their parents arrive for surgery unprepared, stressed, and underinformed. In some cases, the child has not been told why he or she is there and has had no preparation for what is going to happen. In these cases, preparation of the child was left to the parents who did not know how to approach the teaching. The unprepared child is distressed and the parent feels guilt and the normal stress that accompanies a surgical experience.

Pediatric materiel
Pediatric materiel resources are limited in our 14-room operating suite, which serves primarily adult patients. Pediatric supplies are not plentiful, and some are actually scarce. We have two carts with supplies for pediatric anesthesia that are expected to meet our needs. One cart is taken into the room for a pediatric procedure. That becomes a problem if there are more than two pediatric patients. Even when a cart is in the room, a specific item needed may not be available. For instance, the laryngoscopy blades on the cart may be too large and too small, and the desired size is missing. Other items often in short supply are 1-L reservoir bag for ventilating by hand during induction and the right size blood pressure cuff. Pediatric patients vary widely in size and the range of cuffs needed to meet the needs of every patient is quite extensive. This scarcity of supplies results in somewhat of a struggle among the nurses who each want to have everything needed for the pediatric patient in his or her room. The search for appropriate materiel can prolong preparation time, which impacts the flow of the operating room schedule.

Personnel
Pediatric patients are not just small adults. In addition to managing the emotional trauma of a surgical experience, the perioperative nurses must address their unique

physiologic needs and challenges. Perioperative nurses who work routinely with pediatric patients are adept at caring for their young patients efficiently. Caring for only an occasional pediatric patient is stressful for a perioperative nurse whose surgical patients are primarily adults. Nurses want their patient care to be optimal, even under unusual circumstances.

The same applies to the anesthesiologists. HUC has no dedicated "pediatric anesthesiologists." There are some who enjoy being with children, and others who avoid working with them. Every anesthesiologist has his or her own professional style and the nurses must adapt to their unique requirements. Induction of a child can be a peaceful event or just the opposite.

CAN WE IMPROVE?

Not having the resources to provide the best patient care can leave a nurse feeling demoralized and helpless. Being aware of limitations in the environment does not justify sitting around and doing nothing. Professionals meet adverse situations with the resolve to address them and make improvements. According to data provided by the Internal Audit Service, HUC performs 500 surgical procedures on children and adolescents between birth and 14 years of age. Considering that most are accompanied by their parents, it can be concluded that the perioperative nursing staff serves as many as 1500 people in the process of doing pediatric surgery. A group of perioperative nurses at HUC got together to see what could be done to improve the environment and optimize the surgical experience for children, their parents, and their caregivers.

WHERE TO START?

The group began with an in-depth literature search to learn about the rights of children and their unique needs. The rights of children in hospitals are well documented in Europe. The United Nations–approved CRC became the first international law of its type in 1990. Article 38 of the Code of Ethics for Spanish Nurses states that "Nurses in must safeguard the rights of the child." In the American Nurses Association (ANA) Code of Ethics, children are mentioned only as a vulnerable group with special needs to be considered when designing research projects. The CRC speaks not only to the responsibilities of governments, but also defines the obligations and responsibilities of others, such as parents, teachers, health professionals, researchers, and the children themselves. Among the articles in the CRC are the right of children to be heard and taken seriously, with weight given to their views based on their developmental stage, age, and maturity and the right of child and parents to work collaboratively with healthcare providers and to be involved as much as possible in treatment decisions. Of the 23 points delineated in the European Charter on the Rights of Children in Hospital,[1] many are applicable in the perioperative setting (**Box 1**).

A prominent influence on the care of children in health care in Europe is the World Health Organization Task Force for Health Promotion for Children and Adolescents in and by Hospitals.[2] This group targeted the Meyer University Hospital in Florence, Italy, as its prototype hospital. Many countries, hospital systems, and the fundamental mission of the Task Force look to provide scientific support for incorporating concepts, values, strategies, standards, and indicators of health promotion and care for children and adolescents into the organizational structure and culture of the hospital or health service. The Task Force has published excellent documents detailing their recommendations with excellent resources[3] and a template for describing best practices.[4] Many hospitals, healthcare systems, and governments, including the government of the Canary Islands, collaborate with the Task Force and subscribe

Box 1
Elements from the European Charter on the Rights of Children in Hospital that apply to the surgical setting

The European Charter on the Rights of Children in Hospital included as Supplementary Appendix of the European Charter of Rights. Of the 23 rights developed include the following points for possible application in the surgical field:

C. The right to be accompanied by their parents or the person replacing them as long as possible during their stay in the hospital, not as passive spectators but as active elements of hospital life, without that additional costs behave, the exercise of this right should not in any way hinder or impede the implementation of treatments that must be submitted to the child.

D. The child's right to receive information suited to their age, their mental, emotional and psychological status, for the entirety of medical treatment which has been submitted and the positive outlook that this treatment offers.

E. The child's right to a reception and individual monitoring, targeting as far as possible the same nurses and assistants for this reception and care.

L. The right not to receive medical treatment no longer endures suffering unnecessary pain and suffering that can be avoided.

M. Law (and means) to contact their parents or the person replacing them in times of stress.

N. The right to be treated with tact, education and understanding and respect for their privacy.

O. The right to receive, during their stay in the hospital, the care given by qualified staff, who knows perfectly the needs of each age group at both the physical and emotional.

P. Right to be hospitalized with other children, avoiding any possible hospitalization among adults.

Q. The right to have premises furnished and equipped to meet their needs for care, education and games, as well as official standards of safety.

Adapted from European Charter on the Rights of Children in Hospital. Available at: http://www.defensordelmenor.org/legislacion/europea.php.

to its goals. This alliance provided an excellent platform for the HUC perioperative nurses to pursue their quest for improvements.

The Task Force provides a self-assessment tool available to evaluate three areas: (1) the right to optimal health care, (2) the right to participate in healthcare decisions, and (3) the right to protection from all forms of violence.[5] The primary objective in using the tool is to evaluate the actual practices within the facility against the best practices identified by the Task Force. HUC implemented the tool and identified opportunities for improvement. Teaching materials, such as posters based on the Open Letter from Hospitalized Children (**Figs. 1** and **2**), were distributed and improvements were made to accommodate the needs of the pediatric patient throughout the hospital, except for the operating rooms.

The perioperative nurses were determined to take this heightened awareness and commitment to the needs of pediatric surgical patients. They firmly believed that the human factor, individual commitment to improvement, could be the catalyst to overcome the deficiencies in structural design and available resources. The first step was to motivate a change in attitude, behavior, knowledge sharing, skill improvement, and teamwork, and to heighten awareness of the rights of hospitalized children. The improvement project is ongoing and is meeting with success on many levels.

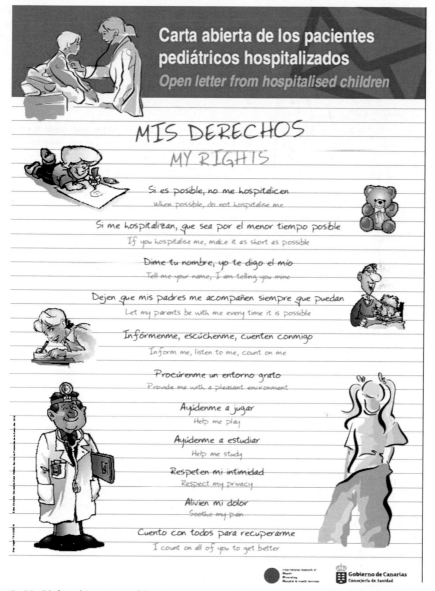

Fig. 1. My Rights. (*Courtesy of* the Canary Islands Ministry of Health. Dep. Legal TF-412/2010. Edita: Dirección General de Salud Pública. Servicio de Promoción de la Salud. Año 2010. Available at: http://www.defensordelmenor.org/legislacion/europea.php; and http://www2. gobiernodecanarias.org/sanidad/scs/content/99c179f0-4a44-11e0-be01-71b0882b892e/Carta MisDerechos.pdf. Accessed September 18, 2012.)

THE IMPROVEMENT PROJECT

To address the child's right to be accompanied by their parents and their right to a safe and pleasant environment furnished and equipped to meet their needs, we adapted a space to accommodate children and their parents before surgery in a room decorated with children's art. There are toys and crafts to entertain the children while

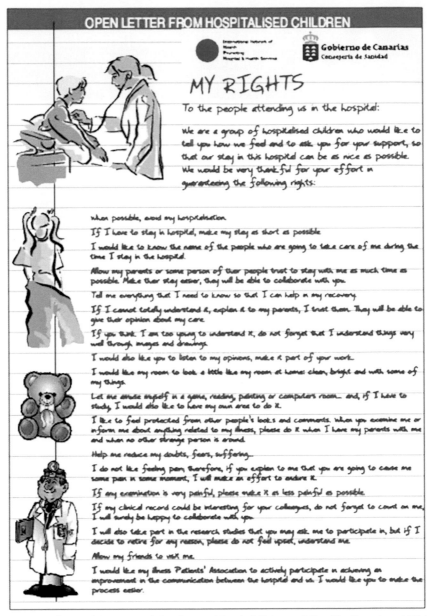

Fig. 2. Open letter. (*Courtesy of* the Canary Islands Ministry of Health. Dep. Legal TF-412/ 2010. Edita: Dirección General de Salud Pública. Servicio de Promoción de la Salud. Año 2010. Available at: http://www2.gobiernodecanarias.org/sanidad/scs/content/99c179f0-4a44-11e0-be01-71b0882b892e/CartaMisDerechos.pdf. Accessed September 18, 2012.)

they wait to be called to the preanesthesia area. The preanesthesia unit nurse involved our pediatric patients in creating the artwork that decorates the room. In support of the right of children to be hospitalized with other children, not among adults, we created a separate section in the preanesthesia area with screens that block the view of the adult patients around them. When possible, parents are allowed to remain with their children in this private space (**Fig. 3**).

In addition to increasing our nurses' aware of the rights of pediatric patients through informal education and inservice, we have ordered the posters and handouts based on the Open Letter from Hospitalized Patients, which will be placed prominently throughout the perioperative environment. It is as important to share this information with children and their parents as with the healthcare personnel. We have also requested the development of educational opportunities for our staff on the various aspects of care of the pediatric surgical patient.

The program needed to address the child's right to be respected as an individual, to receive information suited to their age and developmental status, and to participate in decision-making about their care. This is most effectively achieved by collaborating actively with the children and their parents before surgery and when they arrive in the presurgical area. There are two projects under way to address these needs and the child's right to an appropriate reception and care, as much as possible, by the same caregivers.

We are in the process of creating a pamphlet that describes the surgical experience beginning with arrival into the preanesthesia room, the operating room itself, and the Post Anesthesia Care Unit (PACU). There is a work group designing the pamphlet, which is well-illustrated and written in an engaging manner. The document includes pictures of the environment and the equipment children encounter in preanesthesia, during induction, and in the recovery period. Parents and their children will be able to familiarize themselves with the process and have an opportunity to ask questions and become familiar with the environment before they actually encounter it. There are three parts to the brochure. The first introduces the child and family to the preanesthesia area where they change clothes (if they have come to the hospital from home) and where they might get a mild tranquilizer while they wait for surgery. The second part covers the operating room and what they encounter before they sleep (eg, monitors, blood pressure cuff, pulse oximeter, anesthesia mask, and so forth),

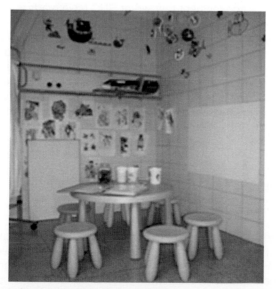

Fig. 3. Waiting room for children and their parents.

so they do not feel assaulted by strange objects. The last part covers the PACU, describing the recovery process and assuring them that their parents will be there at that point.

Our current system of meeting patients for the first time in the preoperative area does not provide sufficient time to assess patient and parent knowledge about the procedure or level of anxiety. We are also planning to implement a nursing preanesthesia visit during which the nurse meets with the patient and parents on the pediatric unit or in the dedicated room for pediatric admissions for those who arrive the day of surgery. At this time, the nurse would be able to assess the child and patient adequately, present them with the pamphlet, and share whatever information is necessary to answer questions and calm their anxiety. When the child and family enter the preoperative area, they will be met by a familiar face; patient and nurse will be more relaxed.

To ensure that the child does not suffer unnecessary pain and discomfort or anxiety, we are also working in partnership with our anesthesiology department to develop protocols for pediatric anesthesia. We are targeting the entire process, beginning with reducing stress in the preanesthesia area, through the surgical experience itself, and into the postanesthesia care unit. Included in the protocol is potential for the administration of anxiolytic medication in the preanesthesia room and the possibility of one parent to accompany the child to the operating room and remain until the child is asleep. Other hospitals that have implemented such protocols report positive results.

SUMMARY

In Europe, children are protected by well-defined rights and laws related to their care. It is important to respect those laws when developing protocols for providing health care for children in our facilities. As professionals, we must be sufficiently informed and educated to provide optimal care and appropriate surroundings. The operating room is one of the busiest and most intense centers of care in a hospital, and therefore one of the most important areas in which to focus on the elements that impact the pediatric patient. One commitment that we at HUC have made is to put protocols in place that improve a child's experience in surgery. Even in a surgical environment that caters primarily to adult patients, it is important to dedicate resources to the care of the children who come to the unit. Even when separate rooms are not available, a small area designed for children can have a positive impact. The protocols must also recognize that the needs of the child and the parents to remain together as long as possible are also important. Age-appropriate, informative literature is very helpful. Like any other specialty, there should be nursing staff with knowledge of the special needs of the pediatric population to give the care, or mentor others who care for the child in surgery. One thing that we were unable to resolve is the need for more pediatric supplies. At this point, we must continue to be diligent in planning for our pediatric procedures and ensure that we share the available supplies so that each child has what is needed.

REFERENCES

1. European Charter on the Rights of Children in Hospital. Available at: http://www. defensordelmenor.org/legislacion/europea.php. Accessed September 18, 2012.
2. International HPH Network. Available at: http://www.hphnet.org/index.php? option=com_content&view=article&id=294%3Ahp-for-children-a-adolescents-in-a-by-hospitals-&catid=20&Itemid=95. Accessed September 18, 2012.

3. The International HPH Network toolbox. Available at: http://www.hphnet.org/index.php?option=com_content&view=article&id=21&Itemid=13. Search Term: "Tool Box". Accessed September 18, 2012.

4. Meyer University Children's Hospital. Health promotion for children and adolescents in hospitals. Official HPH-CA documents. Select "Documentation". Available at: http://www.meyer.it/HPH_NOTIZIA_01.php?IDNotizia=4379&IDCategoria=706. Accessed September 18, 2012.

5. World Health Organization self-assessment tool for pilot implementation. Available at: http://www.euro.who.int/__data/assets/pdf_file/0005/99860/E85054.pdf. Accessed September 18, 2012.

Advocating in Cancer Care

Rebecca O'Shea, MS, RN, OCN, AOCNS, CBCN[a],
Carol Athey, MSN, RN, CNOR[b],*

KEYWORDS

- Oncology • Nursing • Advocacy

KEY POINTS

- Advances in treatment options have made cancer a more controllable disease.
- How the patient and family are told about a cancer diagnosis and how they are supported through treatment and long-term follow-up are critical to adherence and compliance.
- As the number of cancer survivors increases, their unique needs, both immediate and long-term, have become central to nurses' advocacy role.

It is gratifying to see the continued steady decline in overall cancer incidence and death rates in the United States – the result of improved methods for preventing, detecting, and treating several types of cancer.
— Harold Varmus, MD, Director of the National Cancer Institute.

Nurses in all practice settings have a rich legacy of advocacy to uphold. Nurses are ambassadors and patient advocates through each stage along the cancer continuum, from prevention/early detection through active treatment, survivorship, and end-of-life care. Advances in treatment options have made cancer a more controllable disease. After years of dedication to the specialized needs of the cancer population, caregivers are encountering a new normal. How the patient and family are told about a cancer diagnosis and how they are supported through treatment and long-term follow-up are critical to adherence and compliance. Demystifying the fear associated with the word cancer and creating systems that facilitate access to care for all patients will continue to be central to the nurses' advocacy role.

In addition to the prevention/detection and acute treatment settings, there will be a continuous need for survivorship clinics. As more patients survive what was once a more life-threatening disease, new responsibilities emerge. There is a growing population of cancer survivors with complex health care and societal needs, including reduced income and productivity caused by prolonged illness, economic stress, and limited or diminishing social support. In addition, as cancer survivors age, some will be at increased risk for second cancers, requiring additional medical

[a] Texas Health Presbyterian Hospital, Denton, TX, USA; [b] DeWitt School of Nursing Faculty, Stephen F. Austin State University, 5707 North Street, Nacogdoches, TX 75965, USA
* Corresponding author.
E-mail address: atheycj@sfasu.edu

Perioperative Nursing Clinics 7 (2012) 471–475
http://dx.doi.org/10.1016/j.cpen.2012.08.015
1556-7931/12/$ – see front matter © 2012 Elsevier Inc. All rights reserved.

surveillance.[1(p33)] Nurses will help cancer survivors face their significant challenges and rebuild their lives.

Survivors will tell you that a smile, an encouraging word, and a look of support and hope make a difference. Cancer touches all of us in some way. Best practices based on research, evidence, and outcomes must be shared among nursing specialties so that we can support this growing patient population. Education and certification can arm oncology nurses with the knowledge and techniques required to meet their surviving patients' needs.

Nurses caring for this patient population and their families are fortunate to have several professional organizations dedicated to guiding and supporting professional practice at every stage. Without their leadership, nurses would not be the effective partners that they now are in navigating through the upheaval this disease brings to countless lives. The Oncology Nursing Society (ONS) (http://www.ons.org/about) began at the first National Cancer Nursing Research Conference supported by the American Nurses Association (ANA) and the American Cancer Society (ACS) in 1973. After this conference, 4 nurses, driven by a belief that patients and families facing a cancer diagnosis deserved specialized care, started the organization from a garage and a post office box.

The ONS mission is to promote excellence in oncology nursing and quality cancer care; its vision is to lead the transformation of cancer care; and its core values include integrity, innovation, stewardship, advocacy, excellence, and inclusiveness. With 231 chapters and 27 special interest groups, ONS has become a leading resource for nurses around the world. The movement begun by that small group of dedicated nurses who saw a need and took action now includes more than 35,000 registered nurses and other health care providers committed to excellence in patient care, education, research, and administration in oncology nursing. ONS plays an active role in advocacy activities on the local, state, national, and international stage.

The Oncology Nursing Certification Corporation (ONCC; http://oncc.org/About) was incorporated in 1984 as a nonprofit organization that develops, administers, and evaluates programs for certification in oncology nursing. By validating specialized knowledge in oncology nursing and related specialties, it achieves its mission to promote excellence in patient care and professional practice, emphasizing continued competency. ONCC has certified more than 32,000 oncology nurses representing both pediatric and adult populations.

The Nurse Oncology Education Program (NOEP) began in Texas as a grassroots volunteer-based initiative mandated by the then Governor of Texas. Recognizing that educational opportunities were available in the large urban areas of the state but limited in rural settings, the goal was to deliver cost-effective basic information on cancer care to all nurses. It has become hugely successful and a model for similar projects within the United States. Presentations documenting its growth and development have now reached international audiences. Online free continuing education credit on a variety of cancer issues in addition to on-site conferences makes it an invaluable resource for every nurse.

The Texas Nurses' Association/Foundation funds the NOEP, a nonprofit project also funded in part by the Cancer Prevention and Research Institute of Texas (CPRIT) and Live Strong. Based on the motto Every Nurse Can Fight Cancer, NOEP advocates for patients with cancer by providing evidence-based continuing education to nurses with the goal of providing content that will stimulate changes in nursing practice. Education is a powerful tool to promote a healthy lifestyle. Consider that all cancers caused by cigarette smoking and heavy use of alcohol can be prevented. The ACS estimates that, in 2012, tobacco will cause approximately 173,200 cancer deaths.[1(p1)] In addition, scientific evidence suggests that about one-third of the 577,190 cancer deaths expected to occur in 2012 will be related to overweight or obesity, physical inactivity, and poor nutrition, and thus could also be prevented.[1(p4)] The educational activities of NOEP address cancer prevention, detection, treatment, and survivorship. Nurses who pursue education about cancer can use that knowledge to benefit patients, families, peers, and the community throughout their nursing careers.

Advocating: A Team Effort

An oncology clinical nurse specialist (CNS) familiar with options for venous access began work at a community-based hospital where the physicians favored a specific external catheter. Although a multitude of technological advancements were available, physicians consistently selected the external option, with the explanation that "It's working...no need to change or fix"..."That's what the doctor learned how to put in"..."We don't want to stock additional items in central supply."

A staff nurse approached the CNS for consultation and support. She was caring for a young female patient who needed a central intravenous (IV) access line for pain control. Her disease was progressing and the nurse was concerned about her quality of life and supportive care needs. She went on to explain that the girl's passion was swimming. With the customary external catheter, swimming would no longer be permitted. Other nurses joined the conversation, sharing their concerns for this patient whom they had all come to know. With the support of the CNS, they decided to approach the surgeon.

Armed with brochures on various options, they met with the physician. The nurses' enthusiasm captured his attention and his impatience turned to interest as they explained the rationale for an implanted port. The CNS produced a sample device she had previously used for teaching, and, after examining it, the physician asked to speak with the vendor's representative so he could study the technique required to insert it.

Later that week, the internal port was implanted, and the patient was discharged with her pain under control. She was enthusiastic about getting back to swimming. This experience, in which staff from in-patient surgery, education, and the central service department participated, was pivotal in promoting a team approach to problem-solving.

Because of 1 nurse who recognized a patient's need and was willing to advocate for her, colleagues followed her lead. Within months, the team was hosting educational, multidisciplinary in-services house-wide to introduce options. Because of her actions, future patients had choices and physicians recognized and sought out the expertise of oncology nurses. Soon, nononcology nurses were approaching the oncology nurses for support with other patient populations. The oncology nurses became consultants to other areas like the emergency room where nurses called when patients with ports came in. The skill sets involved in managing the devices evolved into a competency in all adult patient care areas.

The success of the nurses' advocacy was highlighted when a patient with an external catheter for antibiotics in place arrived on the Oncology unit. During the discharge planning conference, the nurses realized that he lived alone in a rural community with few resources. In addition, he was losing his sight and could no longer provide his own self-care or afford the needed supplies. Without hesitation, the nurses recommended a port. The surgeon, placed an internal port and the patient went home on schedule. It was obvious that the nurses had been successful in facilitating a change in culture and practice. They had used their knowledge and teamwork to advocate for an improvement that changed outcomes for their patients.

The facility did not have a pediatric oncology unit but did provide general pediatric care. A pediatric nurse approached the oncology nurses explaining that one of his young patients who needed long-term IV access for antibiotics and pain control was refusing an external catheter. The adolescent patient was focused on body image and sports. He had heard about a "lady with an invisible catheter" and was determined to have one. After the oncology nurses had shown him the internal port video, he agreed to having one implanted. The pediatric staff was relieved because they feared he would refuse treatment if no one listened to his concerns.

Sometime later, the device company representative stopped by to thank the oncology nurses for converting the pediatric unit to internal ports. One nurse smiled and replied, "Thank a 13-year-old boy!" He was so pleased with his new port, he managed to spread the word about this option to everyone he knew. That single act of advocacy facilitated more active and normal lives for a population of young patients.

Advocate with Compassion

Simple acts of compassion based on a trusting relationship and knowledge of the disease process and treatment plan can have an important impact on clinical outcomes. Acknowledging, rather than disparaging, a patient's enthusiasm for living, even when her prognosis was poor, may have made a difference in the life of a young woman diagnosed with a late-stage gynecologic cancer. At the time, there were no effective options for many of her symptoms. With little hope for success, treatment was started and the patient put up with tough chemotherapy protocols. Her spirit stayed positive, thanks to the support of family and friends. She explained that she was not only fighting for herself but also for other women who might follow. The nurses were supportive and encouraged her spirit. They marveled at her courage and energy. Her nurse supporters found themselves explaining to their colleagues why this fight was so important to the patient and that she feared others would give up on her because of her advanced disease. When she was discharged, the nurses lost track of her and assumed the worst.

They were astounded when, 5 years later, she was admitted to the oncology unit. Her original cancer was stable and she had been diagnosed with a new primary tumor. She exclaimed to a nurse whom she recognized, "I found the lump myself this time…aren't you proud of me? Thanks to all of you and what you taught me, I caught this one early." Her appreciation for the nurses' support and advocacy on her behalf, even in the face of a poor prognosis, is testament to the impact that advocacy can have on patient outcomes. Nurses never know who their survivors will be; they must support and advocate for all their patients.

Sometimes it is the Patient who Advocates

A nursing student in her senior year was rehearsing her conversation with her parents about how she had made the wrong career choice. Nursing work was hard and her confidence was low. Her love of reading and writing made journalism seem a much more natural choice. She was facing her synthesis clinical; an assignment designed to bring theory and practice together. Her patient was a young boy with a neuroblastoma.

Pediatrics was frightening. She was concerned about the potential for harming a child and the reality of making worried parents more anxious. Knowing little about the disease process of neuroblastoma, its prognosis, or the treatment protocol, she met her patient, a 4-year-old boy wise beyond his years. They bonded quickly and, knowing she was a student, he frequently asked about her homework and whether he could help. Her assignment had been to learn as much about his diagnosis as possible. She explained that she was studying about his tumor and his treatment, but had no idea how it must feel. "I'll tell you," he said.

They sat together and he explained, "I want to get better really fast so my mommy won't cry any more, and my daddy won't be so worried. I don't like lying on that table; it's hard and cold, but my doctor rubs his hands together before he touches me, and I like his warm hands. My favorite nurse in the one who's here when I go to sleep. She holds my hands and tells me stories…and she doesn't even need a book!" The student so wanted to be that nurse; a nurse who could give patient care and tell stories, too; a nurse who could make a very sick child feel safe and hopeful. Sometimes it is the patient who advocates for nursing, and motivates a student to follow a path of learning and caring and making a difference.

REFERENCE

1. Cancer Facts and Figures 2012. American Cancer Society, Inc. no. 500812. 2012. Available at: http://www.cancer.org/Research/CancerFactsFigures/CancerFactsFigures/cancer-facts-figures-2012. Accessed September 26, 2012.

Advocating for the Laryngectomee

Ann McKennis, RN, CNOR(E), CORLN(E)*

KEYWORDS

• Advocate • Laryngectomy • Laryngectomee

KEY POINTS

- Laryngectomy is the surgical removal of the voice box and closure of the pharynx.
- The trachea is sewn to the neck, creating a permanent stoma, which allows the patient to breathe; resuscitation must be accomplished via the tracheal stoma, and oxygen delivered to the nose and mouth goes to the stomach.
- Laryngectomees (those who have permanent tracheal stomas) face challenges in communication, feeding, and appearance.
- Advocating for laryngectomees facilitates a more rapid adjustment to a manageable lifestyle.

A laryngectomy is the removal of the voice box, and the pharynx is closed completely. The trachea, which has been severed, is sewn to the neck, creating a permanent stoma, through which the person breathes. This is the only way that oxygen gets to the lungs. Oxygen and resuscitation must be accomplished via the tracheal stoma. Oxygen delivered to the nose and mouth goes to the stomach.

Laryngectomees (people with permanent tracheal stomas as a result of larynx removal) face major life changes: in their appearance, how they communicate because they are unable to talk, and how they eat. Advocating for laryngectomees facing this difficult challenge facilitates a more rapid adjustment to a different but manageable lifestyle. It is important for patients to know that nurses and patients are partners in care. With the support of nurse advocates, laryngectomee patients can learn to advocate for themselves.

Advocating for laryngectomees includes teaching them and empowering them to teach others about the condition. One of the most important groups to teach is health care providers, who often confuse laryngectomees with people who have tracheotomies. The delivery of oxygen to the nose, occluding the stoma for showering, and resuscitation via mask to the mouth and nose are ineffective, dangerous and life-threatening interventions for laryngectomees. Clearly, there is a need to educate

* 25 Wishbonebush Road, The Woodlands, TX 77380.
E-mail address: mckennis@mac.com

health care providers about the methods that laryngectomees use to speak and breathe. The best teachers are the laryngectomees, who advocate for themselves by teaching the health care providers who care for them. They discuss methods of communication because most providers do not understand Cooper Rand,[1] Servox,[2] Tracheoesophageal puncture (TEP), or esophageal speech. Laryngectomees can explain the method they use, why, and how it works.

They must also share with their health care providers any diet restrictions that they might have. Nutritional support for a laryngectomee can range from needing a feeding tube to eating a regular diet. Humidity is an issue, because a laryngectomee no longer breathes through his or her nose, which normally warms and filters the air; air entering the trachea can be drying. Stoma care is important, normally requiring the use of saline bullets (small vials of sterile saline) or suctioning. The stoma tissue is delicate, and most laryngectomees would prefer to cough up secretions and avoid the trauma of a suction catheter. Providers who see stomas only rarely are often hesitant and uncomfortable with stoma care. Most health care providers are willing learners, and this is the patient's and family's opportunity to make a difference.

Because initially they have lost their ability to talk, keeping a notebook from the time of their initial diagnosis can be helpful for laryngectomees. The journal serves as a history and a tool to review what has worked best. Depression is not unusual for patients who face such a radical change in lifestyle. Medication for depression can help during the postoperative adjustment and the healing process. Pain management is important and advocates should teach the concept of the pain scale so that laryngectomees can communicate well with health care providers. Laryngectomees should carry a medication log that lists prescribed medications as well as supplements, vitamins, herbals, and allergies. Thyroid function needs to be assessed routinely.

Most laryngeal cancers are caused by smoking, and laryngectomees are enthusiastic advocates for a smoke-free environment. Many of them participate actively in health fairs and community projects. They visit schools and talk with the children about smoking and its dangers. Some laryngectomees make routine visits to their legislators and state capitols to advocate for tobacco legislation. Nurses, too, can participate in these same advocacy activities.

There are many resources that are available to healthcare providers that will facilitate their role as advocate to the laryngectomee. Not all cities and states have local support groups for laryngectomees. It is important to make laryngectomees aware of other resources available to them. There are outstanding national support groups that advocate for laryngectomees around the world. One excellent resource is *WebWhispers*, whose primary purpose is to provide practical and educational information and support by way of the Internet to laryngectomees, to all persons diagnosed with or treated for cancer that affects the larynx, or to those who have suffered damage to the vocal cords. Support is directed toward understanding, education, and rehabilitation assistance to be shared with patient, caregivers, and medical professionals.

The *WebWhispers* Web site (http://webwhispers.org/) is a multisection presentation of helpful information that is open to the public. It contains explanations of terms, information about cancer of the larynx, symptoms, treatments, and side effects. There are special sections for before and after laryngectomy surgery. Free information is available to order or download, including choices for learning to talk again, suggestions from vendors, and guidance from health care providers and other professionals.

[1] Herbert Cooper and RAND Corporation, Santa Monica, CA.
[2] Servona, Troisdorf, Germany.

The monthly newsletter, *Whispers on the Web*, contains advice and stories from laryngectomees. One excellent feature is *VoicePoints*, a column that is coordinated and written by professionals for professional colleagues. The *WebWhispers* e-mail distribution list is available only to members (more than 3000, 65% of whom are laryngectomees, and 15% professionals). All members are encouraged to participate to add to the communal knowledge base or to ask questions of the rest of the group.

The mission of the International Association of Laryngectomees (IAL) (http://www.theial.com/) is to support individuals and the families of individuals who have lost their voice as a result of the removal of the larynx. The IAL supports lost chord clubs, assisting and coordinating educational and support conferences. They continue the legacy of 1 laryngectomee helping another on voice issues. They have a quarterly newsletter, an annual conference, and a voice institute.

Support for People with Oral and Head and Neck Cancers (SPOHNC) (http://www.spohnc.org/) is a self-help, nonprofit organization involved in the development of support programs. The organization focuses on meeting the psychosocial needs of patients, as well as preserving, restoring, and promoting physical and emotional health. They publish numerous resources, which include an excellent cookbook, *Eat Well, Stay Nourished*.

The Society of Otorhinolaryngology and Head and Neck Nurses (SOHN) (http://www.sohnnurse.com/) is the professional organization for registered nurses who specialize in otorhinolaryngology (ORL) and head and neck nursing. SOHN fosters the professional growth of the ORL nurse through education and research, as well as providing patient teaching information and professional guidelines.

Dr Itzhak Brook (http://dribrook.blogspot.com) is a pediatric physician, who underwent a laryngectomy a few years ago. He has written many articles that are helpful to the laryngectomee and their families. He is a willing speaker and has presented at numerous professional meetings. His book *My voice: a physician's personal experience with throat cancer* describes his experience and how it has affected his life.

Self Help for the Laryngectomee by Edmund Lauder was written by the father of the current president of The ElectroLarynx Company, who was a laryngectomee. It is often called "the bible for laryngectomees" and at one time was the only resource available. All of the vendors of laryngectomee and voice equipment are wonderful advocates for the laryngectomee.

ACKNOWLEDGMENTS

I thank Pat Wertz Sanders, one of the editors of *Whispers on the Web* for her help and support.

Special Feature Article

Goals for Health Care Reform and Implications for Education and Practice

Deborah Kendall-Gallagher, PhD, JD, RN

KEYWORDS

• Health care reform • Affordable Care Act • Leading change

KEY POINTS

• March 2012 marked the second anniversary of the Affordable Care Act (ACA), landmark legislation designed to transform health care delivery in the United States.
• Understanding how the ACA will impact care delivered in the hospital setting is essential for perioperative nurses if they are to influence and lead change to improve the quality, efficiency, and effectiveness of care.

March 2012 marked the second anniversary of the Patient Protection and Affordable Care Act (P.L. 111–148), as amended by the Health Care and Education Reconciliation Act of 2010 (P.L. 111–152).[1] Known as the Affordable Care Act (ACA),[1] this landmark legislation is designed to transform the current health care system from one characterized by fragmented, uncoordinated care with variable quality, inequitable access, and unsustainable costs, to a system that delivers coordinated, patient-centered care characterized by better quality, better health, and lower costs.[2–8] In addition to expanding access to health insurance,[1] the ACA fosters the development of "clinically integrated, systems-based practice," with the overall goal of improving the quality, efficiency, and cost effectiveness of care using a variety of mandatory and voluntary mechanisms.[6(p.1282)] The ACA provides the framework for transforming the health care system, however, it is the health care providers working at the frontlines of care who actually transform the delivery system.[2,9] Understanding how the ACA impacts hospitals and influences care delivery is essential knowledge for today's perioperative nurse.

This article serves as a primer on the ACA for the purpose of informing perioperative nursing education and practice. The first section provides an overview of the ACA. The second section outlines specific ACA provisions designed to improve the health care

Department of Health Restoration & Care Systems Management, School of Nursing, University of Texas Health Science Center San Antonio, 7703 Floyd Curl Drive, Mail Code 7975, San Antonio, TX 78229-3900, USA
E-mail address: kendallgalla@uthscsa.edu

Perioperative Nursing Clinics 7 (2012) 481–488
http://dx.doi.org/10.1016/j.cpen.2012.08.016
1556-7931/12/$ – see front matter © 2012 Elsevier Inc. All rights reserved.
periopnursing.theclinics.com

delivery system, particularly those that focus on increasing the quality, efficiency, and effectiveness of care delivered within the hospital. The final section discusses strategies and tools perioperative nurses can use to transform their practice within the context of the ACA.

OVERVIEW OF THE ACA

The ACA, signed into law on March 23, 2010, is a comprehensive package of health insurance market and health care delivery system reforms designed to expand access, improve quality, and decrease costs.[10] Close to 1000 pages in length, the ACA includes over 400 different sections organized into 10 topic areas (**Box 1**).[1] The cost of implementing provisions of ACA is estimated at $938 billion over 10 years, which will be financed primarily through savings from the Medicare and Medicaid programs combined with new taxes and fees.[10,11] The ACA is estimated to reduce federal deficits by $210 billion between 2012 and 2021.[11]

The primary goals of the ACA are to increase access to health insurance and improve the quality and effectiveness of the health care delivery system. As outlined in a timeline published by the U.S. Department of Health and Human Services (**Table 1**), provisions of the ACA will be implemented over several years.[1] The government estimates that as a result of the ACA, 32 million Americans who are currently uninsured will have health insurance coverage by 2019 (see Addendum).[10] Increased access to insurance will be accomplished using a variety of vehicles including a requirement that most US citizens and legal residents have health insurance (individual insurance mandate), use of tax credits, expansion of Medicaid, and reform of the health insurance market.[10] Insurance reforms are being phased in over 4 years, with the individual insurance mandate and Medicaid expansion becoming effective in 2014.[1]

To improve the health care delivery system, the ACA uses a combination of approaches including newly created value-based purchasing and innovation in care delivery programs that will be phased in over several years.[1,6] Examples of the multi-year phase-in include educational programs designed to develop the health care workforce (funded in 2010); the new Center for Medicare and Medicaid Innovation created to test new care delivery models (opened in 2011); accountable care organizations (ACOs) designed to encourage integrated care delivery and accountability across providers (effective January 2012); and value-based purchasing programs

---

Box 1
ACA titles

Title I. Quality, Affordable Health Care for All Americans

Title II. The Role of Public Programs

Title III. Improving the Quality and Efficiency of Health Care

Title IV. Prevention of Chronic Disease and Improving Public Health

Title V. Health Care Workforce

Title VI. Transparency and Program Integrity

Title VII. Improving Access to Innovative Medical Therapies

Title VIII. Community Living–Assisted Services and Supports Act (CLASS Act)

Title IX. Revenue Provisions

Title X. Strengthening Quality, Affordable Health Care for All Americans

that link payment to outcomes (effective for hospitals in October 2012 and effective for physicians in 2015).[1]

ACA provisions also reflect the strong support and key role of nursing in transforming the health care delivery system. Several nursing education programs, funded through the Health Resources and Services Administration, were reauthorized and strengthened. Funded programs include the Advanced Education Nursing and Nurse Anesthetist Traineeship programs; the Nursing Student Loan and Nursing Workforce Diversity programs; the Nurse Education, Practice, and Retention Grant program; and the National Health Service Corps.[12] In addition, the ACA funded two practice-related programs, a visiting nurse and social-worker service to expectant mothers in high-risk areas and community-based nurse-managed clinics.[12]

For nurses interested in learning more about health care reform, several web-based resources provide comprehensive explanations of the ACA and its impact on the health care delivery system. Resources include, but are not limited to, the American Nurses Association,[13] the Kaiser Family Foundation,[10] and the federal government's *healthcare.gov* website.[1]

THE IMPACT OF THE ACA ON HEALTH CARE QUALITY AND EFFECTIVENESS

The ACA created a national, multifaceted strategy for improving quality and effectiveness of care using a combination of mandatory and voluntary mechanisms.[6,14] For perioperative nurses, the most pertinent ACA provisions related to quality are those that have a direct impact on hospitals. Belmont and colleagues[6] posit that ACA quality provisions are designed to facilitate "clinically integrated, systems-based care" defined as independent providers such as hospitals or health systems, physician practices, individual providers, and outpatient diagnostic centers that integrate their services through shared electronic health record systems, clinical guidelines, unified practice management, and other techniques. In optimal systems-based care, each patient's health care needs are evaluated and treated as part of a "system" of care for that person.[6(p1282)]

Although the impact of the ACA quality provisions may vary across hospitals because of type of hospital and local health care market,[15] it is important for perioperative nurses to understand the mechanisms within the ACA that motivate hospitals to redesign their services toward clinically integrated, systems-based care. Belmont and colleagues[6] summarized the combination of approaches used in the ACA to drive improvement in quality and efficiency in hospitals as follows:

- "Never-Events" (hospital-acquired conditions): The ACA extends and strengthens the Centers for Medicare and Medicaid Services (CMS) program implemented in 2008 that denies payment for hospital-acquired conditions deemed preventable through reasonable care. Starting in fiscal year 2013, Medicare payments to a hospital will be reduced if it exceeds expected readmission rates. In 2015, CMS will impose an additional 1% annual penalty on a hospital if it is in the quartile of hospitals with the highest "never-events." States must implement "never-event" policies for Medicaid programs or lose federal Medicaid dollars.[6]

- Value-based purchasing: The ACA creates a value-based purchasing program that links hospital quality performance with payment. To fund the program, effective October 1, 2012, hospital discharge payments will be reduced initially by 1% with reductions increased by 0.25% annually until fiscal year 2017. Saved funds will be used to create a value-based purchasing pool that rewards hospitals that perform in the top 50% of comparable hospitals. Performance scores will be based on clinical and patient satisfaction measures. Seven of twelve clinical

Table 1
ACA implementation guide[a] as delineated in U.S. Department of Health and Human Services timeline at http://www.healthcare.gov[1]

2010

Allowing states to cover more people on Medicaid	Prohibiting insurance companies from rescinding coverage
Rebuilding the primary care workforce	Appealing insurance company decisions
Cracking down on health care fraud	Eliminating lifetime limits on insurance coverage
Expanding coverage for early retirees	Regulating annual limits on insurance coverage
Providing free preventive care	Putting health insurance information online
Relief for seniors who hit Medicare prescription drug "Donut Hole"	Extending coverage for young adults
Holding insurance companies accountable for unreasonable rate hikes	Prohibiting denying coverage of children based on preexisting conditions
Providing access to insurance for uninsured Americans with preexisting conditions (high-risk insurance pools)	

2011

Establishing consumer assistance programs in the states	Improving health care quality and efficiency (innovation)
Preventing disease and illness	Free preventive care for seniors
Strengthening community health centers	Improving care for seniors after they leave the hospital
Payments for rural health care providers	New innovations to bring down costs
Prescription drug discounts	Increasing access to services at home and in the community
Bringing down health care premiums	
Addressing overpayments to big insurance companies and strengthening Medicare advantage	

2012

Understanding and fighting health disparities	Reducing paperwork and administrative costs
Linking payment to quality outcomes (Value-based purchasing program effective October 1, 2012)	Encouraging integrated health systems (Accountable Care Organizations)

2013

Increasing Medicaid payments for primary care doctors	Improving preventive health coverage
Increase funding for Children's Health Insurance Program	Expanded authority to bundle payments

2014

Establishing affordable insurance exchanges	Eliminating annual limits on insurance coverage
Increasing access to Medicaid	Increasing small business health insurance tax credit
Helping workers who cannot afford health insurance	No discrimination due to preexisting conditions or gender
Promoting individual responsibility (insurance mandate)	Tax credits for health insurance
Ensuring coverage for individuals participating in clinical trials	

2015

Paying physicians based on value not volume	

[a] See http://www.healthcare.gov/law/timeline/index.html#event20-paneregarding for details of specific provisions.

measures are from the Surgical Care Improvement Project measure set relating to "health care–associated infections, perioperative use of antibiotics, blood glucose monitoring in cardiac patients, venous thromboembolism prophylaxis, perioperative beta blocker use, and, in 2014, postoperative urinary catheter protocols."[1,6,16(C10)]

- Bundled payments: The ACA authorizes a pilot program for hospitals to test the "episodes of care" payment methodology (3 days before admission to 30 days after discharge) for 10 selected health conditions. Covered services include costs for acute inpatient care, physician visits associated with episode regardless of setting, hospital outpatient services, emergency room visits, inpatient rehabilitation, and home health services.[6]

- Accountable care organizations (effective in 2012): ACOs are entities comprised of groups of providers across the continuum of care (eg, hospitals, physicians, and other outpatient providers) that are jointly accountable for care provided to at least a minimum of 5000 Medicare fee-for-service beneficiaries. ACOs that demonstrate savings for the Medicare program, in combination of meeting certain quality benchmarks in 5 domains (patient and care giver experience, coordinated care, preventative health, patient safety, and at-risk populations), are eligible to share the savings with Medicare program.[6]

Collectively, the ACA provisions provide a strategy for hospitals to improve the quality, efficiency, and cost effectiveness of care. Whether or not a hospital can optimize the results as envisioned by the ACA strategy depends greatly on the hospital team's ability to redesign its care processes and form strategic partnerships to deliver clinically integrated, systems-based care.

THE IMPACT OF THE ACA ON NURSING EDUCATION AND PRACTICE

After reading about the ACA, you may ask yourself, "How do I help my unit and perioperative service line redesign its care processes to optimize patient care quality, reduce costs, and contribute to the financial viability of my organization?" This is an important question with a complex answer that merits reflection.

A growing body of evidence suggests that context plays a significant role in the success of quality efforts. In a 2011 qualitative study designed to identify factors associated with better care for patients experiencing acute myocardial infarctions (AMIs), as measured by risk-adjusted mortality rates, Curry and colleagues[17] found that high-performing and low-performing hospitals "differed substantially" in 5 key areas: "organizational values and goals; senior management involvement; broad staff presence and expertise in AMI care; communication and coordination among groups; and problem solving and learning."[(p.384)] The recently developed evidence-based, Model for Understanding Success in Quality, known as MUSIQ,[18] focuses on understanding why, and under what circumstances, quality improvement initiatives work. Many of the factors identified by Curry and colleagues[17] are included in the MUSIQ model. For perioperative nurses actively engaged in efforts to improve quality and reduce costs in response to the ACA, use of the MUSIQ model to guide design of quality improvement initiatives may greatly enhance the probability of project success.

Education of nurses remains a top priority. As evidenced by the ACA, nurses are essential for successful transformation of the health care system. Achieving the goals of the ACA will require interprofessional groups to work collaboratively to develop innovative solutions that eliminate waste in the health care system while improving quality.[19] Continuing to educate current and future nurses, formally and informally, in both the science of improvement and health policy is essential if nurses are to play an influential and lead role in health care reform.

SUMMARY

Efforts to reform health care in the United States are longstanding dating back to the early 1930s.[20] The fact that the ACA is now law reflects broad recognition of the economic necessity for transforming how health care is delivered in the United States. However, the ACA is not without controversy. Legal challenges to the law are currently pending before the United States Supreme Court with the Court's decision expected by June 2012. Unresolved differences among stakeholders regarding fairness in financing (ie, who should pay for health care reform) and ethics of cost containment remain.[21] The challenges to the ACA center primarily on two provisions: the individual insurance mandate and Medicaid expansion.[22] If the Supreme Court finds the insurance mandate unconstitutional, the Court must then determine if the invalidated provision invalidates some or all of the ACA.[22] Notwithstanding the outcome of the Supreme Court decision, the health care delivery system will continue to be transformed in response to economic pressures. The demand for innovative solutions that concurrently decrease costs while improving quality has never been greater.[23] In the words of Linda Groah, Executive Director and CEO of the Association of periOperative Registered Nurses, "An educated nurse is an influential nurse."[24(p17)] Stay informed, be engaged, and influence the process of transformation.

ADDENDUM

On June 28, 2012 the U.S. Supreme Court in a 5 to 4 decision upheld the individual insurance mandate as constitutional under Congress's power to tax. The mandated Medicaid expansion provision was found unconstitutional but severable leaving the other ACA provisions intact. A copy of the full decision can be accessed at http://www.healthcare.gov.[1]

REFERENCES

1. U.S. Department of Health and Human Services. The health care law and you. Available at: http://www.healthcare.gov/law/index.html. Accessed June 1, 2012.
2. Fisher E, McClellen M, Bertko J, et al. Fostering accountable health care: moving forward in Medicare. Health Aff (Millwood) 2009;28(2):w219–31.
3. Kohn L, Corrigan J, Donaldson M. To err is human: building a safer health system. Washington, DC: National Academies Press; 2000.
4. Institute of Medicine. Crossing the quality chasm. Washington, DC: National Academies Press; 2001.
5. Orszag P, Ellis P. Addressing rising health care costs – a view from the Congressional Budget Office. N Engl J Med 2007;357(18):1793–6.
6. Belmont E, Haltom C, Hastings D, et al. A new quality compass: hospital boards' increased role under the affordable care act. Health Aff (Millwood) 2011;30(7):1282–9.
7. Berwick D, Nolan T, Whittington J. The triple aim: care, health, and cost. Health Aff (Millwood) 2008;27(3):759–69.
8. Orszag P, Emanual E. Health care reform and cost control. N Engl J Med 2010; 363(7):601–3.
9. Nelson E, Batladen P, Huber T, et al. Microsystems in health care: part 1. Learning from high-performing front-line clinical units. Jt Comm J Qual Improv 2002;28(9): 472–93.

10. Kaiser Family Foundation. Summary of the new health reform law. Available at: http://www.kff.org/healthreform/8061.cfm?source=QL. Accessed June 4, 2012.
11. Congressional Budget Office. CBO's analysis of the major health care legislation enacted in March 2010. Statement of Elmendorf D before the Subcommittee on Health, Committee on Health and Commerce, U.S. House of Representatives; 2011. Available at: http://www.cbo.gov/publication/22077. Accessed June 5, 2012.
12. Wakefield M. Nurses and the affordable care act. Am J Nurs 2010;110(9):11.
13. American Nurses Association. Health care reform headquarters. Available at: http://www.rnaction.org/site/PageServer?pagename=nstat_take_action_healthcare_reform&ct=1&ct=1. Accessed June 5, 2012.
14. Congressional Research Service. Public health, workforce, and related provisions in the patient protection and affordable care act (PPACA). Available at: http://libguides.law.ucla.edu/content.php?pid=233304&sid=1930567. Accessed June 2, 2012.
15. Berenson R, Zuckerman S. How will hospitals be effected by health care reform? In Timely Analysis of Health Policy Issues (2010). Available at: http://www.rwjf.org/files/research/66028hospitals.pdf. Accessed May 25, 2012.
16. Pritchard D. Spotlight on the centers for medicare & medicaid value-based purchasing programs. AORN Connections; 2012. C10. Available at: http://www.aornjournal.org/article/S0001-2092%2812%2900498-X/abstract. Accessed June 2, 2012.
17. Curry L, Spatz E, Cherlin E, et al. What distinguishes top-performing hospitals in acute myocardial infarction mortality rates? Ann Intern Med 2011;154:384–90.
18. Kaplan H, Provost L, Forehle C, et al. The model for understanding success in quality (MUSIQ): building a theory of context in healthcare quality improvement. BMJ Qual Saf 2012;21:13–20.
19. Martin LA, Neumann CW, Mountford J, et al. Increasing Efficiency and Enhancing Value in Health Care: Ways to Achieve Savings in Operating Costs per Year. IHI Innovation Series white paper. Cambridge, MA: Institute for Healthcare Improvement; 2009. Available at: www.ihi.org. Accessed May 15, 2012.
20. Kaiser Family Foundation. Timeline: history of health reform efforts in the U.S. In Health Reform. Available at: http://healthreform.kff.org/flash/health-reform-new.html. Accessed June 3, 2012.
21. Daniels N, Saloner B, Gelpi A. Access, cost, and financing: achieving an ethical health reform. Health Aff (Millwood) 2009;28(5):w909–16.
22. Noble A, Chirba M. The supreme court on the affordable care act: what are we waiting for. Health Affairs Blog; 2012. Available at: http://healthaffairs.org/blog/2012/06/01/the-supreme-court-on-the-affordable-care-act-what-we-are-waiting-for/. Accessed May 29, 2012.
23. Grant Makers Health. Transforming health care delivery. Why it matters and what it will take. Available at: http://www.gih.org/Publications/StrageticDetail.cfm?ItemNumber=4628. Accessed June 4, 2012.
24. Pyrek K. Innovation, education among the priorities for perioperative nurses. A Q & A with Linda Groah, MSN, RN, CNOR, NEA-BC, FAAN in Infection Control Today. Available at: http://www.infectioncontroltoday.com/digital-issues.aspx. Accessed June 4, 2012.

Index

Note: Page numbers of article titles are in **boldface** type.

A

Perioperative Nursing Clinics 7 (2012) 489–495
http://dx.doi.org/10.1016/S1556-7931(12)00108-8
1556-7931/12/$ – see front matter © 2012 Elsevier Inc. All rights reserved.

self-involvement in, 457–458
surgical procedure examples and, 449–451
Oncology, advocacy in, **471–475**
Oncology Nursing Society, 472
Organizations. *See also* Professional organizations.
advocacy role of, 383–385, 443
Orientation, to perioperative nursing, **437–440**
Outpatient surgery, for older patients, 449–450

P

Pathways to Excellence program, 375
Patient Advocacy Protections Law, 385
Patient Protection and Affordable Care Act, **481–488**
Pediatric patients, advocacy for, **461–469**
barriers to, 462–463
improvements needed for, 463–468
patient rights, 463–467
Peer advocacy, **441–446**
individual, 443–444
organizational, 443
programmatic, 445
programs for, 441–442
Perioperative Nursing Data Set, 426–427
Personnel, for pediatric surgery, 462–463
Prescriptive authority, for advanced practice registered nurses, 369–370, 373–374
Professional organizations
advocacy for, evidence-based practice, 429
advocacy role of, 383–385, **425–432**
AORN, **433–436**
for healthy work environment, 427–428
membership in, 426–427
nursing specialty, **433–436**
certification from, 430
for competence maintenance, 428–429
participation in, 428
Psychiatric disorders, peer advocacy for, **441–446**
Psychological preparation, for pediatric patients and parents, 462
Public events, advocacy at, 390
Public policy
nursing advocacy for, **367–374**
related to elderly persons, 456

Q

Quality provisions, of Affordable Care Act, 483, 486

R

Registered Nurse First Assistants (RNFAs), advocacy for, 373
Research

W

United States Postal Service

Statement of Ownership, Management, and Circulation
(All Periodicals Publications Except Requestor Publications)

1. Publication Title
Perioperative Nursing Clinics

2. Publication Number
0 2 4 4 - 5 3 3 5

3. Filing Date
9/14/12

4. Issue Frequency
Mar, Jun, Sep, Dec

5. Number of Issues Published Annually
4

6. Annual Subscription Price
$132.00

7. Complete Mailing Address of Known Office of Publication (Not printer) (Street, city, county, state, and ZIP+4®)

Elsevier Inc.
360 Park Avenue South
New York, NY 10010-1710

Contact Person
Stephen R. Bushing

Telephone (Include area code)
215-239-3688

8. Complete Mailing Address of Headquarters or General Business Office of Publisher (Not printer)

Elsevier Inc., 360 Park Avenue South, New York, NY 10010-1710

9. Full Names and Complete Mailing Addresses of Publisher, Editor, and Managing Editor (Do not leave blank)

Publisher (Name and complete mailing address)

Kim Murphy, Elsevier, Inc., 1600 John F. Kennedy Blvd. Suite 1800, Philadelphia, PA 19103-2899

Editor (Name and complete mailing address)

Katie Hartner, Elsevier, Inc., 1600 John F. Kennedy Blvd. Suite 1800, Philadelphia, PA 19103-2899

Managing Editor (Name and complete mailing address)

Sarah Barth, Elsevier, Inc., 1600 John F. Kennedy Blvd. Suite 1800, Philadelphia, PA 19103-2899

10. Owner (Do not leave blank. If the publication is owned by a corporation, give the name and address of the corporation immediately followed by the names and addresses of all stockholders owning or holding 1 percent or more of the total amount of stock. If not owned by a corporation, give the names and addresses of the individual owners. If owned by a partnership or other unincorporated firm, give its name and address as well as those of each individual owner. If the publication is published by a nonprofit organization, give its name and address.)

Full Name	Complete Mailing Address
Wholly owned subsidiary of	1600 John F. Kennedy Blvd., Ste. 1800
Reed/Elsevier, US holdings	Philadelphia, PA 19103-2899

11. Known Bondholders, Mortgagees, and Other Security Holders Owning or Holding 1 Percent or More of Total Amount of Bonds, Mortgages, or Other Securities. If none, check box ☐ None

Full Name	Complete Mailing Address
N/A	

12. Tax Status (For completion by nonprofit organizations authorized to mail at nonprofit rates) (Check one)
The purpose, function, and nonprofit status of this organization and the exempt status for federal income tax purposes:
☐ Has Not Changed During Preceding 12 Months
☐ Has Changed During Preceding 12 Months (Publisher must submit explanation of change with this statement)

13. Publication Title
Perioperative Nursing Clinics

14. Issue Date for Circulation Data Below
September 2012

15. Extent and Nature of Circulation

		Average No. Copies Each Issue During Preceding 12 Months	No. Copies of Single Issue Published Nearest to Filing Date
a. Total Number of Copies (Net press run)		291	229
b. Paid Circulation (By Mail and Outside the Mail)	(1) Mailed Outside-County Paid Subscriptions Stated on PS Form 3541. (Include paid distribution above nominal rate, advertiser's proof copies, and exchange copies)	127	105
	(2) Mailed In-County Paid Subscriptions Stated on PS Form 3541 (Include paid distribution above nominal rate, advertiser's proof copies, and exchange copies)		
	(3) Paid Distribution Outside the Mails Including Sales Through Dealers and Carriers, Street Vendors, Counter Sales, and Other Paid Distribution Outside USPS®	4	5
	(4) Paid Distribution by Other Classes Mailed Through the USPS (e.g. First-Class Mail®)		
c. Total Paid Distribution (Sum of 15b (1), (2), (3), and (4))		131	110
d. Free or Nominal Rate Distribution (By Mail and Outside the Mail)	(1) Free or Nominal Rate Outside-County Copies Included on PS Form 3541	59	59
	(2) Free or Nominal Rate In-County Copies Included on PS Form 3541		
	(3) Free or Nominal Rate Copies Mailed at Other Classes Through the USPS (e.g. First-Class Mail)		
	(4) Free or Nominal Rate Distribution Outside the Mail (Carriers or other means)		
e. Total Free or Nominal Rate Distribution (Sum of 15d (1), (2), (3) and (4))		59	59
f. Total Distribution (Sum of 15c and 15e)		190	169
g. Copies not Distributed (See instructions to publishers #4 (page #3))		101	60
h. Total (Sum of 15f and g)		291	229
i. Percent Paid (15c divided by 15f times 100)		68.95%	65.09%

16. Publication of Statement of Ownership
If the publication is a general publication, publication of this statement is required. Will be printed in the **December 2012** issue of this publication. ☐ Publication not required

17. Signature and Title of Editor, Publisher, Business Manager, or Owner

Stephen R. Bushing
Stephen R. Bushing —Inventory Distribution Coordinator

Date September 14, 2012

I certify that all information furnished on this form is true and complete. I understand that anyone who furnishes false or misleading information on this form or who omits material or information requested on the form may be subject to criminal sanctions (including fines and imprisonment) and/or civil sanctions (including civil penalties).

PS Form **3526**, September 2007 (Page 1 of 3 (Instructions Page 3)) PSN 7530-01-000-9931 PRIVACY NOTICE: See our Privacy policy in www.usps.com

PS Form **3526**, September 2007 (Page 2 of 3)